ART THERAPY—the PERSON-CENTRED WAY
Art and the development of the person:

At first Liesl Silverstone thought person-centred art therapy to be relevant mainly for qualified professionals working in the area of therapy. She came to realise that its scope lies in a far wider range of settings.

The book demonstrates this belief. With its many exercises, illustrations and ideas, it is a resourceful manual for

> art therapists,
> counsellors and psychotherapists,
> trainers, teacher, tutors
> social workers,
> nurses,
> occupational therapists,
> youth workers,
> those working with the dyin
> with cancer patients,
> with AIDS sufferers,
> with the abused, with addicts
> the educationally disadvantaged
> with couples, families, teams—

in short, for practitioners involved in the vast field of human development.

Carl Rogers, the course consultant, saw Liesl Silverstone as ploughing new ground. This book could instigate many a new furrow.

ART THERAPY
THE PERSON-CENTRED WAY

Art and the development of the person

Liesl Silverstone

Published in 1993 by
Autonomy Books
17 Cranbourne Gardens
London NW11 0HN

© Copyright 1993 Liesl Silverstone

ISBN 0-9521291-0-8

All rights reserved. No part of this book may be reproduced or transmitted in any form, electronic or mechanical, including photocopy or any information storage and retrieval system, without permission in writing from the publisher.

Reprinted 1994

Manufacture in UK coordinated by Booksprint
20 Shepherds Hill, London N6 5AH

FOREWORD

The world of counselling and psychotherapy is often accused of attaching undue importance to the spoken word as a means of exploring and healing the wounds which life's experience undoubtedly inflicts upon us all. What is more, the therapist who is caught up with his or her own power and authority may be tempted to accelerate the healing process through clever interventions or interpretations which give false illumination and succeed in intensifying the client's confusion or despair. The person-centred therapist, committed to offering empathic companionship rather than expert direction, is unlikely to fall into this trap but may nevertheless often experience the constraints of verbalisation and wish for other modes of accompanying the client on a journey which not infrequently leads to the inexpressible.

Liesl Silverstone's book tells what happens when the person-centred approach is applied consistently to the teaching of art therapy skills. She describes the liberation which her students experience as they learn to acknowledge each other's uniqueness and to share in negotiation and decision-making in a group which treasures the individuality of each member without denying its corporate identity. She shows how new creativity is unleashed as each student discovers his or her own world of images and learns to trust the process of discovery which unfolds as confidence increases. We learn how a group develops in which peer and self-assessment lose their threat and become instead a further spur to self-exploration and enhanced creativity. What is more, we see how students gradually find the courage to take the facilitative approach both to persons and to images into their various work settings and how a transformation can sometimes be effected in clients who have long since been incarcerated in their inner worlds without much hope of change.

In many ways the implication of this book are immense, for it becomes clear that person-centred art therapy as Liesl Silverstone conceptualises and practises it has application far beyond the world of conventional therapy. Her experience points to an invaluable resource for a whole range of professionals working with people and it becomes self-evident that person-centred art therapy would constitute an admirable component in almost any training course where human suffering and human development are central issues.

Liesl Silverstone benefited from the guidance of Carl Rogers in the early days of her training work. Liesl's contribution, then, is firmly anchored in the tradition of therapy which trusts the client's resources and has every confidence in the client's capacity to find his or her own way forward. Through her own patient application of this affirming philosophy to the realm of art therapy she has extended immeasurably the terrain which is now accessible to those who may never previously have stumbled upon the treasure-house of their own healing imagery.

Brian Thorne
Norwich, 1993

To Pat Milner,

who has encouraged me consistently on my path,
with my appreciation, admiration, and love.

Acknowledgments

I am indebted:

to Dr Kenneth Gray for his interest and initiative in getting the course certificated by Crawley College,

to Stuart Milner, Principal of Crawley College, for his constant help and goodwill,

to Brian Thorne, for his support and understanding, made manifest in the title and foreword of this book,

to David Brazier, Charles Merrill, Tony Merry and Robin Shohet for their help-full feedback,

to Sheila Dainow, for all manner of assistance,

to my sons Daniel and Robert for their interest and encouragement,

to numerous past students for their contributions, and, above all,

to the students of the course for their willingness, honesty and enthusiasm in sharing so much of themselves; for breathing life into the book.

Contents

Introduction	i
The Course	xvii

AUTUMN TERM: 1
The Person-centred Approach

SESSION ONE — 3
Introductions: using art to break the ice
- Exercise WITH IMAGE (1) 'Me now' — 6
- Exercise 1: Sharing hopes, fears, expectations — 7
- Exercise WITH IMAGE (2) 'Me in the group' — 7

SESSION TWO — 11
The person-centred approach: about Carl Rogers Empathy, acceptance, congruence. A listening exercise. Using art to re-connect with memories about being/not being heard.
- Exercise 2: A name game — 11
- Exercise 3: Listening in pairs — 13
- Exercise WITH IMAGE (3): Listening — 14

SESSION THREE — 18
Reflecting. The victim/persecutor/rescuer triangle and art, to uncover blocks to empathic listening.
- Exercise 4: Reflecting the visual — 19
- Exercise 5: Reflecting — 20
- Exercise WITH IMAGE (4): Victim/Persecutor/Rescuer — 22

SESSION FOUR — 25
The blame—placate—generalise—distract—level model, and art, for further work on blocks to empathic listening. Counselling practice
Practice in threes: Counsellor/Client/Observer
- Exercise 6: A teacher you liked/disliked — 25
- Exercise 7: Role play: Blame/Placate/Generalise/Distract/Level — 27
- Exercise WITH IMAGE (5): Image re Blame/Placate/Generalise/Distract/Level — 27
- Exercise 8: Listening in threes: Client/Counsellor/Observer — 28

SESSION FIVE	33
Acceptance—using art to identify the origin of non-accepting beliefs	
Exercise 9: A secret	33
Exercise 10: Non acceptance	34
Exercise WITH IMAGE (6): Least acceptable behaviour	34
Exercise 11: Counselling practice in threes	36
SESSION SIX	42
Projection	
Exercise with image	
Half-term review	
Exercise 12: Reflecting in the round	43
Exercise 13: Projection	43
Exercise WITH IMAGE (7): Guy Fawkes	45
Exercise 14: In pairs: Half Term review	47
THE DAY	51
Students negotiate and produce their contract and assessment procedures.	
Personal sharing with image	
Exercise 15: Drawing up the group contract	52
Drawing up the assessment procedure	53
Exercise WITH IMAGE (8): Life line	53
SESSION SEVEN	61
Books, Congruence	
Exercise 16: 'I' Statements	64
Exercise 17: 'I'm least congruent when—'	64
SESSION EIGHT	68
Sharpening up group contract. Clarify personal contract	
Counselling practice	
Exercise 18: Counselling practice in whole group	69
SESSION NINE	77
Attitudes re assessing/being assessed	
Exercise WITH IMAGE (9):	78
Guided fantasy re assessment	
Exercise 19: Discarding unwanted messages	81
SESSION TEN	85
Feedback	
Exercise 20: Voicing paranoid fantasies to group members	86
Exercise 21: Giving/Receiving feedback	86
SESSION ELEVEN	91
Personal Contracts finalised	
Exercise 22: Ratifying personal contracts	91

SESSION TWELVE	99
Dealing with unfinished process	
SESSION TWELVE that-might-have-been:	105
End of term 'games'	
Exercise 23: Boasts	105
Exercise 24: Love game	105
Exercise 25: Giving/Receiving positive feedback	105
Exercise WITH IMAGE (10): Gift giving	106

SPRING TERM: 111

Bringing the person-centred approach
to art therapy

SESSION THIRTEEN	113
The creative process	
Theory—Exercise re creativity—Exercise with image	
Exercise 26: Messages re creativity	120
Exercise WITH IMAGE (11): New Year	121
SESSION FOURTEEN	130
Guidelines for the person-centred facilitator	
Exercise with image	
Exercise WITH IMAGE (12): an animal	137
SESSION FIFTEEN	143
More experiential learning	
Exercise with image:	
Exercise WITH IMAGE (13): A rose bush	144
SESSION SIXTEEN	150
Guided fantasy	
Exercise WITH IMAGE (14): A costume room	150
SESSION SEVENTEEN	157
More practice	
Exercise WITH IMAGE (15): Magic Gift Shop	157
SESSION EIGHTEEN	162
Person-centred supervision	
Valentine's Day	
Exercise WITH IMAGE (16): a Valentine card	166
SESSION NINETEEN	168
Imaging without a theme	
Exercise WITH IMAGE (17): Circle walk	169
SESSION TWENTY	173
Fairytale	
Exercise WITH IMAGE (18): Once upon a time	173

THE DAY	178
Individual and group work with images	
Exercise WITH IMAGE (19): Group island	179
Exercise WITH IMAGE (20): Mother	182
SESSION TWENTY-ONE	186
Using an existing image. A taster of Gestalt	
Exercise WITH IMAGE (21): Tarot: Counsellor/ Client dialogue	186
Exercise 27: Symptom dialogue	188
Exercise 28: Parent dialogue	189
Exercise 29: Eating a biscuit	189
SESSION TWENTY-TWO	192
Art Therapy and Gestalt	
Exercise WITH IMAGE (22): Guided fantasy: Motorbike	192
SESSION TWENTY-THREE	197
Use of person-centred art therapy with small groups	
Exercise WITH IMAGE (23): Small groups: draw a house	197
Exercise 30: End of term summary	199
Exercise WITH IMAGE (10): Gifts	200

SUMMER TERM 205
More practice
Self/peer assessing of portfolios and certificating

SESSION TWENTY-FOUR	207
Working with the whole image-making process	
A guided fantasy	
Exercise WITH IMAGE (24): deep sea diver	209
SESSION TWENTY-FIVE	212
Working with the whole image-making process	
A guided fantasy:	
Exercise WITH IMAGE (25): Wise old person	213
SESSION TWENTY-SIX	218
First Portfolio Exchange	
A group exercise with image	
Exercise WITH IMAGE (26): Symbol in the round	220
SESSION TWENTY-SEVEN	224
Second Portfolio Exchange	
Another group exercise with image	
Exercise WITH IMAGE (27): Group Mandala	225

SESSION TWENTY-EIGHT 234
  Third Portfolio Exchange
  Incorporating Art Therapy, 'on the hoof' in a counselling session
    Exercise WITH IMAGE (28): Introducing art therapy 'on the hoof' 234
SESSION TWENTY-NINE 240
  Assessment/Certificating
MODERATOR DAY 249
  Course moderator meets the students
    Exercise WITH IMAGE (29): Getting out of a box 253
SESSION THIRTY 256
  Ending
    Exercise WITH IMAGE (30): Stocktaking 259
    Exercise 31: Angel Cards 261
APPENDIX I—One year on: The student's comments: 267
  'What I am doing differently at work as a result of the course.
  How I have changed as a result of the course.
APPENDIX II—Some students from other groups comment. ... 273
APPENDIX III—More recent students' work settings. 287
BIBLIOGRAPHY 289

Introduction

Several years ago I went to Czechoslovakia, the country of my birth, with my son.

In Prague, we visited the Jewish museum. There, in the section about Terezin—the concentration camp where all my family were sent before being deported elsewhere—I saw a collection of children's art: with the most meagre material available, children had expressed, in images, how they felt to be in Terezin.

The seeds of my work with art therapy, of this book, were sown during that visit.

I was trained as a social worker; to solve the client's problem, to know best. I was well accustomed to that model since childhood—someone telling me what to do, what not to do. Now, as an adult, it was very easy to perpetuate the model. I knew of no other.

Then, as a student on a counselling course, I came across the approach of Carl Rogers; the person-centred approach based on the belief that the person knows best, and can reach her own potential in a climate of acceptance, congruence and empathy. Emotionally I discovered the benefit for myself, from the client's chair: to be heard empathically, to be deeply understood; that kind of listening felt like a precious gift where, in turn, I could trust listening to myself. To be accepted, unconditionally, without judgment, enabled me to look at the unacceptable aspects of myself, to work through and go beyond them. To experience the counsellor as real, genuine, congruent, encouraged me to trust her and, in turn, let myself be real.

Intellectually I embraced this approach at once and with enthusiasm. It made abundant sense on many levels—personal, social, political, international. Yet it took me a very long time to integrate, to operate. The old authoritarian model had to be uprooted first.

Slowly I began to see the benefits in my work as a school counsellor, extending the person-centred approach to young people, watching their self-esteem grow. And yet, and yet—I began to note the limitations of mere words, began to search for some other mode of knowing.

Images. Art therapy. I discovered first (inevitably) for myself the power, the potential, the truth contained in images made visible. I trained as an art therapist. I learned that images, like dreams, tap into the world of spontaneous knowing, nothing to do with thoughts. When dialoguing with a picture I'd have those moments of 'aha!' when the image gave up—or rather, I recognised—a message to me. Through art therapy an integration between the thinking and the knowing mode, between conscious and unconscious material, could take place. I brought the person-centred mode of facilitating to the world of art therapy—allowing the *client* to know what the picture meant. No interpretations. No guess work. No me knowing best. The evidence was astonishing, encouraging.

I offer courses, based on experiential self-discovered learning in person-centred art therapy, training people working with people.

As counsellor, I introduce art therapy whenever appropriate.

Slowly, based on my enthusiasm about this harmonious marriage of the person-centred approach and art therapy, the idea of a book took shape. How? What to say? Would words reduce the experience, the essence of the 'now', the magic of the image? I procrastinated.

Then, during the first session of the certificate course, one Wednesday afternoon in September, an enormous 'aha!'. I know: I will record, on the hoof, one year's course, this group's course, using the students' *own* discoveries as evicence: discoveries in becoming person-centred, in exploring their world of images, and in applying person-centred art therapy both on the course and in diverse work settings; immediate, alive, dynamic, not me reporting 'about'. So: a truly person-centred book. I am excited. I share my idea with the students. They agree to participate (all but one). We have a 'book file' and each week students can add their contributions, their perceptions, difficulties, discoveries. I set myself a regular weekly writing slot. And so, quite naturally, in its time of readiness, the book emerges.

The seeds sown in the museum of Terezin are bearing fruit, transforming tragedy from the past to a health enhancing resource for the here and now.

So much for my stepping stones.

Now to the course—the vehicle for passing on my discoveries in book form, the symbolic illustration of the journey on the road to person-centred art therapy.

Prior to the course, prospective students come to a selection evening. I tell them about the philosophy and format of the course, so that they might know clearly, what to expect.

Similarly, in this preface, I offer such a summary, that the reader might be better prepared to embark on the journey alongside the students of this book.

Firstly, the person-centred approach.

Carl Rogers himself evolved his theory through self discovery. That is to say, he did not formulate an intellectual theory then to be applied to people. Rather, he found from his interactions with—initially—clients, that the person has the capacity to know best.

This, the core of his theory.

He discovered that three basic conditions were required to create a safe climate within which such knowing could occur:

1) Empathic listening—the ability to offer the fullest attention to the client. When the client feels herself truly heard and deeply understood, she may hear herself truly, and feel trusting enough to explore further.

2) Acceptance—extending unconditional positive regard, a non-judgmental attitude to the client. When the client knows that all of her is accepted unconditionally, she may in turn accept all of herself, and move on to discover what she may become.

3) The capacity to be honest, open, congruent with the client. When the client sees the counsellor as genuine, she too may trust herself to be genuine, enabling her to move and grow.

This, then, the theory of the person-centred approach in a nutshell, the nut to be cracked and examined in detail during the course.

The theory is concise. The practice has led to the largest amount of documented evidence of any therapeutic approach, showing its effectiveness in personal development, that growth, integration, and a more autonomous way of being can ensue, at every level of development.

The theory is so easy to understand intellectually, so difficult to incorporate into one's way of being. Very few of us have experienced a model in our unbringing which is based on the belief that the person knows best. So, it is like learning a new language. During the learning, the old language will keep getting in the way.

Carl Rogers said of this course: 'It is based on a philosophy which empowers the person and helps to make them more self-directed.' That is indeed the aim and scope. And I need to recognise at the outset that most of us resist owning our power, becoming self-directed. We've been used too long, to be told by others what to do, and more often, what not to do. This has led us to believe that we are incapable of knowing for ourselves. We collude; we ask others what's best. We give up our power to parents, teachers, employers, the clergy, politicians—all those who profess to know best for us.

On the course—a microcosm of society—I aim to reverse this process. A student will ask me a question. I'll say: what do *you* think? The student can then discover that she knows the answer within herself. She has re-claimed a little of her power, has begun her journey towards becoming person-centred.

I remember myself, as a student on a student-centred counselling course, feeling outraged, that first term, having to make my own decisions. Why can't the tutor tell me what to do—that's what a proper tutor does. I nearly left. My heartbeat quickens at the thought—of missing what became for me my watershed. So, on the course, I can empathise very well with those who, initially, struggle with the person-centred approach and all it implies. I need to remember, very humbly, that I'm a mere step or two ahead, that I can fall into old ditches when the going is rough.

For most of us it is hard to come by the three basic attitudes, because we ourselves had not been listened to empathically, had not been loved unconditionally, and had not experienced genuineness in others.

The necessary learning does not occur through reading about, writing about, talking about—the criteria of traditional education—but through much personal work. Firstly, we need to discover what gets in the way of being person-centred. Old automatic strategies learned in childhood need to be identified. Only after such—often painful—uncovering, can we relinquish the old, be available to the new. So we spend much time during the first term, with much use of images, on such uncovering before we can begin to be empathic, accepting and genuine, before we can begin to extend that way of being to others. This can be a slow and painstaking process.

The course structure is based on self—and peer—assessment, underscoring the central belief that the person knows best, and giving the students the possibility to put the belief into practice.

Throughout the course the students give one another feedback. In this way they can become more congruent, and moreover, flatten the authoritarian pyramid by sharing power. In the autumn term the students devise their own group contract and assessment procedures. They decide what to learn, when and how to bring evidence of such learning. The final assessing is to say whether a student has gained the certificate —or not. The students themselves take responsibility. The students themselves know best. This, the political aspect of person-centredness: how to be self-directed within society, how not to give up personal power to leaders. Students have the opportunity to empower themselves, to discover how difficult this can be and to apply the experience in other settings.

I am committed to the person-centred approach. I have experienced its benefit for myself. I offer it as a counsellor, and as a trainer. I know that personal development can occur in a climate of acceptance, empathy, genuineness. I know when an individual is regarded as trustworthy and responsible, she/he can move towards a more autonomous way of being. So why add another component—art.

Through research conducted mainly at the California Institute of Technology by Roger Sperry, the separate functions of the two hemispheres of the brain were revealed, showing that each hemisphere perceives reality in its own way. The mode of the left brain is thinking, analytic, judgmental, verbal; the right brain non-verbal, spacial, spontaneous, intuitive, creative, non-judgmental. Sperry says: Modern society discriminates against the right hemisphere. In education, science and the work-place, academic knowing, rather than intuitive knowing, is favoured as a selection criteria, a value-judgment.

In therapy—a microcosm of society—it can happen that by talking about, the client can stay in his/her left side of the brain, and not connect with repressed material on the right side of the brain—the very material needed for integration. By introducing imaging, made visible in art-form, and working with it in a person-centred mode, that integration can occur.

Images contain messages from the subconscious—perhaps hopes or fears—needing to be known. Alice Miller writes: 'the spontaneous images I began to do helped me not only to discover my personal story but also to free myself from the intellectual constraints and concepts of my upbringing and my professional training.' When thoughts are pushed aside, spontaneous images can emerge: symbolic aspects of the self, in need of recognition.

During the second and third term of the course we focus on such images, such recognition. There are four stages:

1) Imaging—allowing images to present themselves to the inner eye;

2) making those images visible in art-form;

3) trying to elicit the meaning of the image with a person-centred facilitator;

4) working on the emerging issue in counselling.

Let us look a little closer at each of these steps:

1) To aid the shift from the thinking to the creative mode, a theme or a guided fantasy can be a helpful vehicle. Whilst imaging, we aim to push aside censoring, judging, thinking. It is possible to illustrate a thought, but then you simply illustrate something you already know, and you are unlikely to learn anything new.

Allow an image to come up, without censoring, without thinking. Trust it; let it come. The more you can say 'I have no idea what this image is about' the more likely it is to be about a great deal. On the course the students experience a large variety of imaging exercises. They discover for themselves how to relinquish thought, trust the image, and tap into their right-side brain.

2) Simply the process of externalising the image to art-form, illustrating some event or feeling can, in itself, be healing. The picture releases, expresses and contains within

a manageable boundary hitherto repressed material. A child painting a thunderstorm can connect with her fear of thunderstorms in a safe way and feel lighter as a result. Edith Kramer, an art therapist working with children, says: 'Forbidden wishes and impulses can be symbolically expressed. Painful and frightening experiences that had to be endured passively can be assimilated by actively reliving them on a reduced scale.'

3) Buber says: 'To become an I, I need a thou.' And so it is with images. The client can get further, talking about the picture with a counsellor. A person-centred counsellor. One who does not interpret, know best. Violette Oaklander, a gestalt art therapist working with children, says: 'I believe there is no way you can make a mistake if you have good will and refrain from interpretation and judgment. Most of us have good will. Few of us refrain from judgments, or even notice that we are interpreting.'

It is easy to embrace the person-centred approach intellectually. However, much personal work and practice is needed to eliminate old ingrained patterns—such as the need to be needed, to know best, to control, to solve the problem, to impress—before one can shift towards being truly person-centred. The students engage in such work on the course.

There are purists who define person-centred counselling as a process confined to words. The image is a projection of the self, made visible. Thus, when incorporated into the counselling dialogue, the meaning of the symbolic aspect can emerge, and contribute significantly to the therapeutic process. As with words, the person-centred counsellor respects the ability of the client to know for herself. As with words, the counsellor's task is to hold the mirror up, in this case to the picture, and to the client's process in creating the picture, to allow the client to see—or not to see.

The danger to identify and interpret is even greater when working with images, because of their powerful emotive impact, and awareness is needed to push one's own reactions aside, to be available to the client only.

Maslow says: 'Creating tends to be the act of the whole person. He is then most unified, most integrated. In moments of here and now we don't reject or disapprove, we become more accepting. Spontaneity allows the honest expression of our whole uniqueness.' The person-centred mode, so akin to the creative mode, both being nonjudgmental, accepting and existential, makes for a harmonious partnership.

4) The image can release its gift quickly. That is not the end of the story. The gift, brought to awareness, may need to be worked on in counselling. This may take rather longer: 'I saw a strong serene tiger. What I drew is a fluffy cuddly pussycat.' The client cries. She cries that she keeps her tiger hidden, and shows only her cuddly pussycat. Insight within minutes. Now she needs to explore ways of making her tiger visible.

On the course students have ample opportunity of imaging, and eliciting the meaning of the image from 'client' and 'counsellor' position, as well as from the 'observer' role, in giving feedback.

The person-centred counsellor needs to develop a shift of focus to incorporate three new aspects in working therapeutically with art:

1) The mirror is held up not only to words, but to the picture.

The counsellor may reflect the whole process of image-making, not only the end product:

'You took a piece of paper and folded it in half.'
'You started, turned the paper over, started again.'
'You tore a piece off.'

The size/colour of paper, material used, may be reflected:

'You took a large white sheet.'

'This is the only part you did in red.'
Position, size:
'You put yourself on the edge of the page.'
'What about the size of this shape.'
That which is missing can be significant:
'I notice there are no hands.'
'You have left this part blank.'
Wider reflections can be fruitful:
'You drew mother in red paint, you in grey chalk.'
'Last week you used only black, this week there is no black.'
All these elements, however unawarely chosen by the client, can be of importance.

2) The picture is an extension of the self in symbolic form made visible. Therefore the facilitator needs to help the client towards recognition of such projected material by making 'bridges' from the picture to the client. However well you work with the picture, if you treat it as something separate from the person you are not working to full effect.
'I need to define the shape of this cat.'
'Does that speak to you? Defining the shape of the cat?'
'Oh yes! I need to define *my* shape! *Me*!'
'I'm puzzled. I'm terrified of the violence of these men.'
The bridge here took the client to a denied childhood memory.

3) In 'eye to eye' counselling, not everything the client says needs to be reflected. When talking about an image, the client becomes less self-conscious, and the words he/she uses become ever more spontaneous and uncensored. Words become 'right side of the brain' words of potential significance. These the client needs to hear. Thus it can be that more words need to be reflected when working with images.
'I couldn't bear to draw the image, it disturbed me so much; these three black roses.'—These spontaneous words

lead to denied feelings about the three children who have left home, and the client's changing role as mother.

Sometimes the whole process needs to be reflected, as a re-enacted symbolic microcosm:

'It took you a long time to get into the water; you're very afraid of it; you need to make sure your oxygen cylinder is in position. Then you swim to the bottom of the sea and discover a treasure in the cave.'

Sometimes noting that which is missing, leads to a shift: Pam is twelve. Her mother has died. She does not talk about it—she is cheerful. She draws her house; her bedroom, with Pam in it; her brother in his bedroom next door, bathroom, living-room with father and girlfriend. 'No kitchen' I say. Pam cries: 'That's where mum used to be cooking, talking to me...' The dam has burst. She could grieve, let go.

At every level of development, the therapeutic use of art releases and enables shifts in awareness and development.

A trainee at an occupational training centre for mentally and physically handicapped adults, who lives in a hostel, draws a picture of a bride and groom—she and John—and talks about her wish to be married. The next week she makes a collage of washing machines, furniture, food, garden—all that makes a home. Again, she talks about her wish to be a home-maker with John—safely contained in art-form. The following week, an abstract zig-zag of her anger. She gives voice to her frustration, her rage about her limitations, her handicap. Initially, she did not think she could make pictures. As well as expressing her feelings, she tapped into her ability to be creative, enhancing her confidence.

We are born creative, even though our culture may not value creativity. With art we can rediscover our creative force which releases such an amazing array of symbolic images. They come to us, bearing their gifts. And a person-centred counsellor can help us recognise such gifts. Somehow, by thinking less, it is possible to know more.

Working with art is, in itself, a creative spontaneous process, as the counsellor moves from words to image, to feelings, to body language, to wider reflections. Wherever the focus of the moment, counsellor and client proceed on a journey into the unknown, a magical mystery tour.

Counselling with the therapeutic use of art is most scopeful: imaging can be suggested 'on the hoof' during a session, to explore further a feeling, a situation, an emotive word.

A woman talked about her friend who had promised to ring her the previous night, and did not do so. She felt disappointed, abandoned. I suggested she close her eyes and let an image come to her to do with 'abandoned'. She drew a baby in a cot, crying, a wall, and a woman the other side of the wall turned away. She spoke of herself, the baby, and the mother who never came when she wanted her. She was amazed. A memory from pre-verbal times. Thus far all her work in therapy to do with issues of inclusion and exclusion, had not brought up this memory. The image connected her to the source of her belief in herself as being unloveable, as someone to be excluded, to her exclusion of herself.

Images can go back even further. A woman comes, unable to understand her anxious feelings about belonging. Her own memories produce no connection. Imaging around her anxiety, she draws a foetus in the womb. She, in her mother's womb. Mother, newly arrived from Europe, fleeing Nazi persecution. The foetus imbibing mother's anxiety about belonging.

A couple came to look at their relationship. During the first session they draw a 'conversation' on paper: one makes marks on one side of the paper, the partner on the other. A space in between. Two sets of marks in their separate territories, never touching. This is an exact illustration of their relating: our contract, made visible. During the last session, the picture was much more balanced, the two colours inter-twining, together and separate, both.

So, not just for individuals, but for pairs, families, groups.

Art is a help-full language for those less able to express themselves verbally. It can be equally relevant for the articulate, who can use words to distract, defend and delay.

I have worked with a selective mute; we dialogued with images, to reach a point when the client selected speech.

Unlike words, which we can forget, the picture keeps. We can refer to it, know at once what it means, relate change to it. A safe and accurate way to share intimate discoveries.

At every level of development, person-centred art therapy releases and enables shifts in awareness and integration. It is applicable in a variety of settings: working with the terminally ill, with AIDS sufferers, the abused, the addicted, the bereaved. Imaging symptoms, feelings, hopes and fears can all lead to release and reconciliation. Nurses, occupational therapists, teachers, youth workers, managers, as well as counsellors and therapists, have discovered the benefits of including imagination, creativity and art as a means to knowing the whole person.

Often students come to the course, initially, to gain a certificate. By the time they leave they tend to report that the chief benefit has been the amount of self-awareness they gained.

They could uncover two aspects which may have been dormant within themselves: the capacity to be person-centred, and the key to their image world. And they can combine the two. Now they can take their learning to their diverse work settings.

I hope that the reader, in following the students on their journeys of discovery, might similarly be able to make relevant discoveries for himself/herself.

The book is a manual, with many ideas and exercises. And it is more than a manual. The students of this group have breathed life into the book. In sharing with the reader their feelings, hopes and fears, the drama and the dynamic of their interactions, they illustrate in an immediate and personal way how it is to move from the familiar to the new, to encounter obstacles on the way and to report the delight at their hard-fought-for evidence and insights. What better way of showing the value of person-centred art therapy than by their self-discovered learning, making this a truly person-centred book.

It is my hope that ever more counselling courses may incorporate the creative therapies, of which art is one, in their training programmes as an invaluable means towards integration and growth. In turn, more art therapy courses might benefit by including the person-centred facilitative approach on their syllabus.

As I developed the training course, I discovered that imaging can be used to great effect in learning. For example, we may be looking at acceptance. The students list the behaviours they can least accept. I suggest they close their eyes, and, with their least acceptable behaviour in mind, go back in time and see if an image, a scene, emerges to do with this behaviour; and sure enough, they re-connect with the source of such non-accepting feelings. They can then reclaim the projection, and become more accepting. Creativity in education.

The person-centred approach, at first developed in counselling, then was seen as relevant in a far wider range of settings: education, management, family, religion, politics etc. Perhaps similarly, the person-centred approach linked to creative modes has relevance in a wider field. Integrating the intelligence from both right and left sides of the brain could bring about the ability to function more fully. Surely this is beneficial to persons, wherever they may be. What an exciting notion! Imagine!

For now, you can read on and see how to come by art therapy the person-centred way.

Liesl Silverstone
London, 1993

REFERENCES

Roger Sperry, *Lateral Specialization of Cerebral Function in the Surgically Separated Hemispheres*. In F.J. McGuiguigan and R.A. Schoonover eds., *The Psychophysiology of Thinking*, N.Y. Academic Press, 1973. p.vi.

Alice Miller: *The Drama of being a Child*, Virago Press 1987. p.vii.

Martin Buber, *I and Thou*, T & T Clark 1970. p.viii.

Abraham Maslow, *Therapy and the Arts*, edited by Walt Anderson—Harper 1977. p.ix.

Violette Oaklander, *Windows on our Children*, Real People Press 1978. p.viii.

Edith Kramer—*Art as Therapy with Children*, Feder. p.viii.

The Course

"I have come to feel that the only learning which significantly influences behaviour is self-discovered."

Carl Rogers

Purpose

That the students themselves come to discover their difficulties and successes in becoming person-centred, in exploring their world of images, and in bringing the person-centred facilitative approach to the image, both on the course and in their diverse work settings, as a means towards healing, self-awareness and growth.

That they come to see person-centred art therapy as a valuable teaching aid, to reinforce, deepen and integrate their learning, understanding and insight.

For easier reference, all exercises in the book are printed in italics.

When making general observations, the author uses 'he' or 'she' with the definite intention of including all persons.

Permission to quote the table on page 113 from Drawing on the Right Side of the Brain *by Betty Edwards has been granted by Souvenir Press Ltd, London.*

AUTUMN TERM
The Person-Centred Approach

Purpose for whole term

To enable students to understand the theory, experience for themselves, and offer to others the person-centred approach, focusing on its three main corner stones: empathy, acceptance, congruence.

To pave the way, students will have the opportunity to become aware of old behaviours which prevent being person-centred.

The learning will be reinforced, helped and deepened with the use of images. Thus, students will experience the power of images in the process of learning itself—a key component of the course—and see its relevant application in other educational settings.

Every component will be based on experiential learning, the students finding out for themselves. There will be ongoing self and peer assessment throughout. Students will draw up their own group contract (what they are agreeing to learn) and assessment procedure (how they will demonstrate their learning), culminating in their certificating procedure. This, a key experience of person-centred negotiating, power-sharing, decision-making.

Students will see the relevance of all such experiential learning in other settings and take opportunities to apply it. Students will be encouraged to read relevantly, to be clear about theory.

The tutor teaches, models, clarifies, brings her in-sights and experience.

SESSION ONE
Introduction

"Every person born into this world represents something new, something that never existed before, something original and unique. Every person's foremost task is the actualisation of her/his unique, unprecedented and never recurring potentialities, and not the repetition of something that another, and be it even the greatest, has already achieved."

from *Reform Synagogue Prayer Book*

Purpose

This session is about the coming together of thirteen strangers, how to allow that process:
a) Giving names—'what I do';
b) deciding on practical issues: smoking, confidentiality, dates, time to monitor—allowing group 'norms' to emerge;
c) giving clear outline of the course: this is what we're here for;
d) opportunity to express hopes and fears in pairs: make one 'friend';
e) say: 'this is me' with an image;
f) say: 'this is me in the group'—with an image—and so, the first discovery of using images.

We arrive. Twelve women. One, away on holiday, will join us next week.

We sit around the room, shoeless, on floor cushions—to help us be at ease. Each one says her name and what she does—her 'label':

Dawn: a residential social worker with children;

Heather: a teacher in a family therapy unit;

Wendy: a co-ordinator for cancer support group;
Geraldine: a Relate counsellor;
Marianne: a counsellor for people with drink problems.
Rosemary: a voluntary worker facilitating art groups in a mental hospital;
Kim: a teacher working with groups of children;
Helen: a volunteer worker with the elderly;
Nina: an educational social worker;
Jo: a photo therapist;
Mary: the absent member, a staff nurse, working with the terminally ill;
one student—a family therapist. Initially this student did not want to be named in the book. Later, she agreed to being referred to as 'a student'.
and I, the course tutor;

I am excited by the mix, by the diverse possibilities of applying the course work.

We deal with 'housekeeping'; smoking, lifts. We negotiate the term dates. We agree on ten minutes' monitoring time before the end of each session:...time to record, make notes, on the content of the session, on personal insights, group process etc. We define confidentiality: that anyone, on leaving the group, can talk about anything that is personal to herself; she cannot, however, disclose anything about other group members. We agree to adhere to this formula.

I clarify that the focus is on training rather than therapy; learning is by doing, personal material *will* emerge and can be explored within a limited space of time. Some students may find that they need to take such material to individual counselling, for further exploration.

I say something of my role as a person-centred tutor: you have agreed to come to learn about person-centred art therapy, and we have two hours per week for 30 weeks. So I see it as my responsibility to prepare a structure to cover the ground. Within that structure, there will be scope to negotiate, alter, omit and propose. This is how I see myself holding the balance, within our time limit, between suggesting and negotiating.

Then something of the proposed course format: the focus in the first term will be on the person-centred approach, using images to aid the learning process. We will work in groups of two, three, four, the whole group—whatever seems appropriate. Learning will be based on self and peer assessment throughout; this entails giving one another—and oneself—honest, caring feedback after each exercise. Attendance is, therefore, important on two levels: the student is present for her own learning, and also, to take responsibility for observing and giving feedback to her peers.

On the whole day of the autumn term, we will spend the morning working out a 'group contract'—*what* we have agreed to learn together—and the assessment procedure—*how* we will demonstrate that learning. From this contract each student will produce her personal contract, to be ratified by peers, saying how she, in her individual way, in her personal work setting, will fulfil the group contract. Thereafter, each student will know clearly what material to incorporate in her portfolio to be brought in the summer term for assessment. This is a very crucial experience for the students: how to take responsibility for decision making.

Person-centred education in action. Very different from the traditional model, where authority figures—tutors, directors of education—decide on course criteria, on assessment procedures, the student the passive participant.

I explain the role of the course moderator, who spends the day with us all in the summer term. She is the bridge between Crawley College and us. She will check out that the procedures we've devised, and the manner in which we've implemented them, are of a standard, show a level of responsibility, good enough to warrant the College awarding its certificate to this course. In a way, the students become their own education authority. We are modelling something new. The person-centred approach in educational, political terms. An invaluable experience of the course.

In the afternoon of the Autumn Term day we will do an art therapy exercise as a group.

During that term I will show my books. It is important to me that students read 'about', *after* they've experienced for themselves; that they might read Rogers and be able to say: 'Yes, I know, I've discovered this for myself.' Person-centred reading.

The focus on the next two terms will be on art therapy exercises, facilitated in a person-centred mode. The day of the spring term will be spent on an individual and a group art therapy exercise.

Jo asks if it's OK for her to take photographs during the sessions—

We move on:

Exercise with image (1)—'Me Now'
I suggest the students close their eyes, focus on how they are feeling.
 'Without thinking, let an image emerge, a symbol, of you, now. When you're ready, open your eyes, and convey this image.' Then, each student says her name, talks about her image:

'This is a droopy flower. I feel rather droopy today.'

'I'm a foetus, curled up in this bubble, waiting, hoping, to uncurl, to emerge.'

'This red box is my anxiety. On top of it, this green and blue is my hope, my excitement'. *See Fig. 1.*

'These are bubbles of excitement, anticipation.'

'This green bit is reaching out, this dark blob is unsure, stuck.'

I suggest they note the quality of the two 'name' exercises; the one saying her name and what she does, and the one using an image to describe herself.

The second enabled sharing with the symbolic language of images at a feeling level, quickly, safely, accurately. Within the first hour of the group's life.

Exercise (1)—sharing hopes, fears, expectations
We did an exercise in pairs. Each partner took five minutes to focus on her hopes, fears and expectations of the course. Each partner gave some feedback to her listener as to the quality of her listening. The first opportunity for a taster of congruent feedback.
Each student then introduced her partner to the group.

We shared how that was; anxieties about 'getting it right', hiccups in the listening process, the joy of having someone's attention, making one contact in a new group.

Exercise with image (2)—'Me in the group'
I placed a large sheet of paper on the floor.
'This sheet represents the group. Now put your symbol on the sheet to reflect how you feel in the group. Take your time. Adjust it if you want—how near, how far, to whom.'
Each woman then spoke of her position on the page:
'I'm a bit off the page, a bit on—that's how I feel.'
'My fear of covering someone else's work conveys so clearly to me how much I hold myself back—I musn't be too pushy, I must stay in the background.'
and the student whose image was thus covered—'but that's just how I feel; I need to hide a bit.'

I am struck by this example—how often with images, made spontaneously, there is accurate evidence about interconnecting.

I suggest, the students note how, with this exercise, they were able to illustrate familiar strategies, to share issues about relating.

It is monitoring time. During this time students will be able to record what they learned about the person-centred approach, about art therapy, about themselves. We've broken the ice. I look forward to next week.

Comments

The course takes place in a large room of my house. I need to be clear of my territorial boundaries.

Before the session I experience a mixture of feelings: excitement, apprehension, a touch of resistance.

Excitement—a voyage into the unknown! Another group of people with the opportunity to discover that which I hold dear: person-centred art therapy. Another possibility for me to do that which I am committed to, enthuse about, do well: the teachings of person-centred art therapy.

Apprehension—will we get on? What are these people like, these twelve people who I don't know? Will I be up to it, be spontaneous enough, notice and deal with whatever manifests itself in an open, caring, helpful way, or will I become automatic? Will my enthusiasm carry me away? Will I be liked?

Resistance: In June I separated from three course groups. By June much closeness, warmth and trust has been established; the ending is not easy—a real loss. The price of working in a way where it becomes safe to share, be intimate. Am I ready to embark on such a journey again? Will I hold back, to avoid closeness?

It's a bit like waiting for a party to begin, waiting for the guests to arrive.

They arrive. In no time at all I forget my apprehension. Let the party—as if for the first time—begin.

Two students have left behind their pictures. What are they, symbolically, saying? What, of themselves, do they not want to take away? Not just our words, our entire process—verbal, non-verbal, aware, unaware—has meaning. During the year, we will have the opportunity to focus on, integrate the non-verbal, the unaware.

I think we achieved our purpose of coming together. (I realise, when I am clear of the purpose, I am likely to offer relevant material). Students have been able to discover for themselves how, with an image, it is possible to express feelings more easily, safely, accurately, than with the use of words, thoughts, only. They were able to share more about themselves, in a group of strangers, than in other settings.

There were no judgements, interpretations. Comments were accepted for themselves. Bringing the person-centred approach, and the image, together. A microcosm of the course to come.

Already, in this way, some degree of trust, of safety, emerged, for some of the students.

It is said that, often, the comments made by the client in the first five minutes of the session are crucial.

It occurs to me that here is a parallel:

Comments students made about themselves, as they placed their image on the group space, were issues which re-emerged throughout the year.

And for me, this was the session when I decided to write the book!

I recall, when writing my paper on person-centred art therapy, I needed—as required by academia—to find quotes in other people's books, to say what I want to say. I wrote to Carl Rogers, asking for a booklist on person-centred art therapy. He replied that he knew of no such books, that it seemed to him I was ploughing new ground—ever since when I've had the knowledge that I would write such a book. Slowly I've been nudging myself towards this, gathering evidence, expertise, confidence, focusing on the structure; that I would record a course group's process, thus illustrating person-centred art therapy in action, not only me writing about, but others reporting for themselves.

I realise that the 'trigger' for me to feel: 'Yes, this is the group'—was Jo's offer of contributing photographs—for I'd been resisting the solitary task of writing—now I'd have some help. After the session I spoke to Jo about the idea of the book. She seems to like the principle. Next week I will share my plan with the students.

Paradoxically, Jo stopped taking photographs—for her it was a means of staying in 'observer' position; she needed to take more active part. But by then I was under way. Jo's offer was sent to me, to get me going.

Application

It is hoped that the reader will transpose and apply the session's material as appropriate to his/her own situation.

Each week I am giving some relevant examples under 'Application'. Thus, this week, an exercise as an 'ice-breaker', a safe way of saying: 'this is me'.

Any group meeting for the first time—courses, training, support groups, teams, staff groups, classes etc.

SESSION TWO
About Carl Rogers—listening exercises
—the book

"Such listening as this enfolds us in a silence in which at last we begin to hear what we are meant to be."

Tao Te Ching

Purpose

To include the thirteenth course member.

To get to know each other's names.

To give the theory of the person-centred approach, as originated by Carl Rogers.

To offer an exercise for empathic listening and to discover blocks to such listening.

To offer an exercise with imaging, to fetch the student back to the cause of such listening blocks.

To show the power of intuitive knowing, through the image, which leads to valuable awareness.

To plan for book-contributions.

We welcome Mary into the group.

We fix the term's dates: beginnings, endings, half-term, the whole day.

Exercise (2) A name game
We play a 'name game'. We stand in a circle. I say my name—pause—and throw a ball to a student. She says her name—pauses, so that her name be heard—throws the ball on. When everyone has said her name at least twice, the rule changes: the student throwing the ball calls out the name of the person to whom she is throwing the ball. We stop, after some two turns each.

I outline what I suggest for today: I want to say something

about Carl Rogers, and then, to offer some exercises around listening. The group members agree.

It is important for me to suggest, rather than decree, the proposed content, to allow room for students to negotiate, adjust, change. The person-centred mode in group action.

They have come to a course on person-centred art therapy; that is the given content. Within that agreed syllabus, there is room to negotiate, whenever relevant—as we shall see.

Now, to Carl Rogers: He came to therapy from theology. He made his discoveries based on his inter-actions with people—rather than developing a theory in laboratory-like conditions, then to be applied elsewhere. He found that the person knows best, that if we do not interfere—advise, correct, criticise, praise—then the person might move towards his/her fuller potential. He found that a certain climate was necessary for such development to occur. Such a climate required three basic attitudes:

(1) Empathic listening. Total listening, leaving yourself aside, being fully available to the other. When you are offered such listening, it is as if you are receiving a precious gift. And yet such listening is hard to offer—it is not a model most of us experienced in our upbringing. Much work is needed to weed out old patterns, to be able to listen in this way.

(2) Acceptance. Unconditional positive regard. Truly accepting the person, as he/she is at that moment. Non-judgementally. If I criticise, you will need to defend yourself, you will not be able to explore that which I criticise. If I accept you, you may feel safe enough to look at the issue you bring, to work through it, move on. Again, a difficult approach to offer as my own prejudices, my own conditioning of being judged, intrude. Again, much work is required before I can become truly accepting.

(3) That I be genuine, congruent, not pretending, wearing a mask. If I am genuine, you may learn to trust me. If I am phoney, you will pick it up, hold back.

If I can listen empathically to you, in time you may learn to listen empathically to yourself. If I accept you totally, in time you may accept yourself, your dark aspects, the total you. If I am genuine, you may become congruent, honest with yourself.

It is like learning a new language, for most of us were taught another language, based on conditional love. So we will do exercises here to help us discover the old obstacles, before we can learn the new language.

More of these three corner-stones anon.

Briefly, something about Roger's developmental model: a baby, every baby, wants love. Slowly the child discovers when she gets love, when not. 'I will love you if...you are quiet, go to sleep, are clean, do well...': conditional love. Slowly, the child modifies her behaviour. She is dependent, needs love. Slowly, she denies aspects of herself to gain approval, love. Perhaps much later, in therapy, she might reintegrate those denied aspects, and the feelings that went with the need to deny—anger, rage, pain. Most of us were reared in such a system. Alice Miller calls it 'the poisonous pedagogy'.

So, it is not enough to want to be Rogerian, person-centred. We have to unlearn, undo much old imput, before we can become person-centred. The model offers a total shift of power; if I stop controlling you, you may become autonomous.

To me, real power is, when I feel OK in myself, in touch with my own power, I can sit back and let you have yours. Anything else is control. So, I have to work hard to feel OK in order to sit back, be person-centred, allow you to become.

Exercise 3—Listening in pairs
I suggest an exercise, in pairs, each person to listen for five minutes to the other. They get into pairs:

'Notice your body language. Is your body saying: I am paying you my fullest attention'—some adjust their position. I say that the speaker share something about herself, take responsibility for the level of sharing—today, and in all ensuing exercises. The listener simply to listen, not speak, perhaps notice what goes on for her as she listens.

After five minutes the listener tells her partner what went on for her. Partner may want to respond. They swap over, and share again.

Then they share in the group:

Jo doesn't like silence.

Marianne identifies with her partner—several others nod.

Geraldine needs to ask questions, to be helpful.

Rosemary interprets, gives meaning.

Wendy is unsure of eye contact.

I distribute a 'handout' on empathy and focus on blocks to empathy—i.e. defensiveness, need to be liked, needed, expectations—which lead to non-empathic behaviour—i.e. judging, interpreting, identifying, information seeking, looking for solutions, reassuring. All these behaviours distract from the ability to listen totally, to pay undivided attention. Students discover that 'simply' to listen is not simple at all; much gets in the way of empathic listening. Much nodding, as students recognise their own blocks, and ensuing behaviours.

Exercise with image 3—Listening
I say something like: 'close your eyes. Focus on the exercise, we've just done on you listening, perhaps on what you noticed about you not listening fully. (Pause) See if an image comes up for you. A scene. (Pause) Maybe from now, or an earlier time. (Pause) Now convey that image to paper.'
They do. Then each person says something about the image.

Jo's picture is of a locked door. She's alone, can't bear silence (makes a link with the listening exercise when she didn't like silence), needs to justify herself. She says: 'No-one listened, so I have become what I wanted others to be for me.'

Kim does an image of large eyes, trying hard to get it right for parents—whilst her stomach in knotted. She says: 'I was trying very hard to listen to Wendy. This reminded me of always trying very hard to do well, especially academically'—so she goes into overdrive. Tries too hard and, paradoxically, doesn't hear at all.

Nina draws a wire mesh—'No-one heard me the other side. I realise that my need to listen to others springs from a need to have been listened to—sometimes it is the next best thing to get for myself, by providing it for others.'

Heather draws a house and garden. She is by herself. She says: 'In my image of an empty but friendly house, that is what I felt tuned into. The people around were on another wavelength.' *See Fig. 2.*

Dawn draws a picture of herself listening to other people's problems. No-one had time to listen to her own problems, so she must always get it right for others, to avoid the pain of her own problem, and of not being heard. Catch 22.

Geraldine needs to be very helpful, do more than her share, give advice.

Wendy draws a shut door—no-one there when she needed them—earlier she was unsure about eye-contact—having got none. When Jo speaks, Wendy identifies—takes the focus to herself—one way to be heard. *See Fig. 3.*

With the image, each woman seems to recall how it was as a child NOT to be listened to. The message is: you're not worth attention. Self-esteem stays low. The ensuing strategy: perhaps I can exist by being there for others. A non-person-centred stance.

We can see that with words, teaching about/learning about/talking about empathy, we reach one level; the image helps to reach deeper levels, helps to make links, awarenesses, with an immediacy and a truth which is visible, cannot be readily denied.

I note again how the sharing of personal issues, through

images, helps to establish trust—even after two sessions. The students learned about empathic listening—not as a skill, a theory, but on a very personal level of discovering.

There was sadness about, recognising how little of empathic listening was modelled to us as children. We learn strategies by which to survive, wise strategies for a child. The question is: how helpful is it to perpetuate such strategies for life? Students begin to see that much work is needed to recognise, to shift such unhelpful strategies in order to be free to empathic listening. They see how the imaging exercise leads to such recognition. Imaging as a tool in teaching and self-awareness.

I give a handout: the word 'to listen' in Chinese.

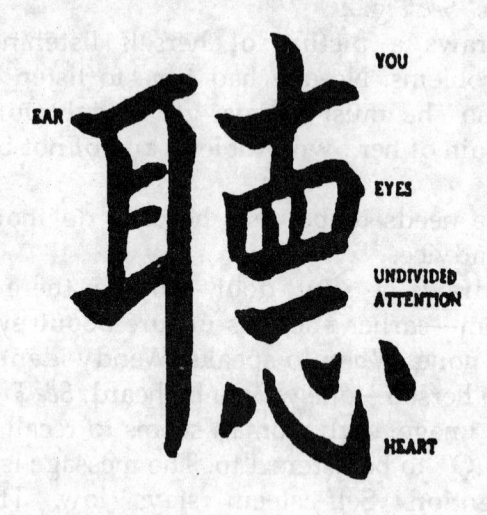

聽

EAR
YOU
EYES
UNDIVIDED ATTENTION
HEART

Now I tell the group my excitement about writing the book. I hope that each week they might want to contribute some of their written discoveries, their evidence—to make the book truly person-centred. I suggest that each person decides on the use of her name—real of pseudo—by which she be called in the book.

There is a sense of excitement in the room—everyone

agrees that the basis of the book be about this group, this year.

Later Helen says: 'I felt like a cog in an important wheel, part of a dream, to be involved in Liesl's book. I felt a surrendering into the whole year's situation—much less feeling of separation than in the first week.'

Comments

It seems valid, in experiental learning, to lay the foundations with input of theory. The house, then, is built.

This week, the students discovered between them for themselves all the blocks to empathic listening mentioned in the handout. Now they know—the handout reinforces.

The art exercise connects them, swiftly, accurately, to the cause of such blocks—how they developed strategies to do with not being listened to themselves. Only with such awareness can the cultural chain be broken, can something new occur.

I realise, in remembering my own journey on the person-centred road, that not all that long ago I was where the students are: unable to listen emphatically, with numerous old defences getting in the way.

(Like: 'Let me give you the answer, then my invisible parent will see what a clever girl I am, approve of me. And you will be impressed, need me.')

Application

Any course teaching counselling, therapy, art therapy, inter-personal skills.

Any course in education wanting to incorporate art and imaging as a learning aid.

Any group wishing to further good communicating.

In short, any person wishing to convey the message to another: I hear you, I understand you, I respect you.

SESSION THREE
Reflecting
Victim/Persecutor/Rescuer triangle
using art

"I see him through his eyes."

Sufi saying.

Purpose

The purpose of this session is to continue with empathic listening in a more active way: how to reflect back what a person has said, to paraphrase. I demonstrate, the students practice. They have an opportunity to discover:

(a) How it is to be listened to so completely;
(b) how it is to offer such listening, and
(c) what gets in the way.

In order to illustrate a model more familiar in our culture, I describe the 'victim', 'persecutor', 'rescuer' triangle. Sometimes, in order to move on, first we need to know what stops us moving on, remove the obstacle. With the use of an imaging exercise, each student can get in touch with the position of the triangle most familiar to her, and where, in her story, it belongs/originates. On offer: more evidence of the value of images, as against words.

The list of students' addresses is handed out. One student says she does not want to contribute to the book. She would add bits, but the book would be mine, 'like the man who just impregnates, but the woman carries and produces the baby.' Later, she says I may refer to her as 'a student'.

I go on to talk about reflecting: it is 'simply' (only it's not so simple) holding the mirror up to the client—reporting, without interpreting, judging, identifying, knowing best, that which you hear.

Exercise 4—*reflecting the visual*
*In pairs, two minutes each way—with feedback in between:
As 'counsellor', simply reflect what you see, as if you are the mirror—client stays silent—i.e. 'your head is turned to the left side, your right hand is holding your left hand.'*

In the feedback, several people needed to interpret—i.e. 'you are relaxed', 'you are tense'. Heather becomes as her 'counsellor' wants her to be: She hears: 'You look tense'. She thinks: 'she must be right—I better look tense.' Geraldine is embarrassed to be noticed. Helen feels awkward to have the spotlight on herself—learning in the 'client' chair.

I go on to talk about reflecting: not a total parrot—like action-replay, rather, a summing up of the essence. Paraphrasing, using metaphors, are creative ways of reflecting. Always reflect feelings—the mountains in the landscape—the crux of counselling. If you get feedback that you avoid reflecting feelings, consider what that's about for you—what are *you* avoiding? As we progress, voice, expression, body posture are reflected. As we get more familiar with the process of real listening, making wider reflections is helpful:

'You say you are worried, and you are laughing.'

'Every time you talk about your father, you shut your eyes.'

The client hears herself reported back accurately, feels truly heard, gains trust and clarity, and is able to go further.

So much for the basic ingredients. I will add others to the recipe as the cooks become more experienced.

I suggest, I'll demonstrate for five minutes.
One student volunteers:

Dawn: 'I've reached a watershed.' (Laughs.)

Liesl: 'So you've reached a watershed, and you laugh.'

D: 'It's no laughing matter. My relationships have been a kind of crutch to me. Now I want something different, to be separate. And I'm scared.'

L: 'You've had partners for some kind of safety. Now perhaps you want something else, to be on your own, and you're frightened.'

D: 'Yes. I haven't any guidelines to tell me how to go. I need to know what I want, and not operate on 'shoulds'.'

L: 'You may need to make your own decisions, based on what you want rather than what you ought to do, and you have no model to go on.'

D: 'Yes. I have a few wordless clues deep inside, what I want.'

L: 'You have an inkling, a feeling in your gut about your needs.'

D: 'Yes. I must listen to myself more.'

Feedback from Dawn: 'I have a need to *hear* myself asking for help, as I've never been able to do it *directly* before.

I liked the paraphrasing—it didn't sound mechanical. I felt heard, and reinforced, and was able to say more. Most people don't hear, and I need to say it again and again. Yes, it was good.'

She has discovered for herself how it feels to be truly heard: the outcome of empathic listening.

Exercise 5—Reflecting
The students work in pairs.
For the first five minutes, one is 'client'—talks about herself; the other is 'counsellor'—listening, reflecting. Then the 'client' gives the 'counsellor' feedback.
They swap roles for the second five minutes, again giving feedback.

Back in the whole group, an opportunity to share:

Helen notices she can't take a silence, needs to come in. Needs to explore what her discomfort is about.

Much happens in silence. As in winter, when much goes on underground, unseen. The counsellor needs to allow that process—and note how she stops herself allowing it.

Marianne is nervous of 'interrupting': in reflecting, you are NOT interrupting; simply saying the client back to the client. Often this feeling of interrupting comes from conditioning of 'little girls should be seen and not heard'. I have no right to interrupt, focus on me.

Several students report the need to interpret, to ask questions.

In wanting to become person-centred it is very important, first, to discover one's own difficulties, and to deal with them. As the course is a training course, needing to cover a specific syllabus, only some time can be given to personal work. And this could well mean, having one's own counselling, support group, supervision, time and space to focus on the self—away from the course.

So, first, from the client's chair, to listen to oneself, discover and accept the self, to be truly genuine about oneself, and *then*, only then, to offer that opportunity, as counsellor, to a client. And this may need to be an on-going process. Rogers talks of the counselling encounter being a meeting of two imperfect people, one of whom, for a period of time, is in the role of counsellor, the other, client.

I share one formula towards self-awareness: Four stepping stones:

(1) Unaware incompetence. (I don't know I'm not listening fully).

(2) Aware incompetence. (I know I'm identifying).

(3) Aware competence. (I know I'm listening to you fully now).

(4) Unaware competence. (I'm listening to you as naturally as breathing.

I talk about the model of:

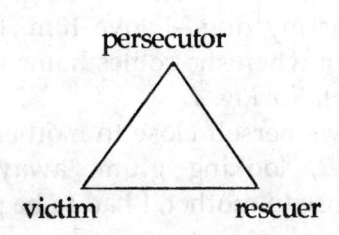

persecutor

victim   rescuer

The rescuer goes: oh, you poor thing; let me do it for you. The persecutor wags her finger, criticises. The victim says: I'm too helpless to manage on my own. Poor me.

Both rescuer and persecutor keep victim in victim position. There is collusion between the positions. 'V': please help me. 'R': of course. 'P': you're useless.

Sometimes the only way to get noticed is to be in victim position. Even to become ill. *'Then* she'll pay me attention'.

All positions are controlling. We can whizz round the whole triangle: I persecute you (P), I feel guilty and need to make reparation (R), I feel sorry for myself that I can't get it right (V).

None of these positions are person-centred. Persecutor judges, rescuer solves the problem, victim gives up her power to others.

Exercise with image 4—Victim/Persecutor/Rescuer
I say: 'Close your eyes. Reflect on these three positions—rescuer, persecutor, victim. (Pause). Maybe one speaks to you more than the others. (Pause). Now, let an image, a scene, a picture surface, about these positions. (Pause) Maybe from long ago. (Pause) Who is doing what? (Pause) What about you?—What do you feel?—How old are you? (Pause).
Now, open your eyes and put your image on paper, however you want.' We decide to share in the group, to help us form as a group.

Rosemary draws a man persecuting her, she then persecutes the dog. She says: 'Mother is out at work. This man comes to look after me, persecutes me in all kinds of ways. I don't know how to stand up to him. I'm angry. I hit my dog. I don't want to hit my dog—I love him. I feel confused. I can't tell my mum when she comes home from work.' (Kick the cat syndrome). *See Fig. 4.*

Geraldine draws herself close to mother, father behind a newspaper, sister, looking glum, away from her and mother. 'To be close to mother, I had to be good. Father kept out. Sister was the clever one. To get noticed, I rescued.' She cries. 'I didn't get to this in therapy. I'm sad about myself.'

Heather draws herself getting in the way. *See Fig. 5.*

Marianne draws a small fist clutching a hankerchief. 'I'm victim. I get persecuted by my sister. I feel all alone.'

Nina draws a large black shape, and smaller shapes in mauve. 'This (the black shape) is mother, and this (mauve) is us—the rest of the family. Mother persecuted me. In my teens, I persecuted her back, though it wasn't what I really wanted to be doing.'

Jo draws herself, drowning, one arm up. The other arm stretched out to rescue. She calls the picture: 'Dying to save somebody else.' *See Fig. 6.*

Most of us have very little experience of being truly heard. We hardly know how it is to be deeply understood. We perpetuate what we did experience, emulate what was done to us. So the business of listening to someone totally, is hard to come by. And only after diligent personal work, uprooting old behaviours.

So, we are reinforcing our learning with images this term, helping us to discover blocks to being person-centred. I cannot be empathic, accepting, congruent, whilst in the Victim/Persecutor/Rescuer triangle.

I am glad some students have started contributing to the book file:

Kim writes: 'The VPR triangle has sparked off many personal images of violence, isolation, drowning, goodness as a survival mechanism, opting out—things not ready to be dealt with. This was moving.

I admired 'a student' today, who said 'no' to contributing to the book. She seems to have such courage to stand up and say 'no'. I would so like to be able to do that.'

Geraldine: 'I was amazed how much, and at what depth, could come up with an image in such a short time.'

Comments

Some students expresss surprise at the amount of self-awareness gained with the help of an image made visible. So much so soon.

Regarding the student who does not want contribute to the book, I wonder: during the summer, this student sent me an essay about her use of art in her work, (the images were illustrations of her analytical thoughts, not images in the true sense). She wanted my comments. I declined, as I felt this would skew the group dynamic even before we began. I said I would be pleased to discuss her paper during the year. Was her unwillingness to participate now, some response to this?

Today, the topic 'reflecting': as tutor, I like to reflect students' comments to them, as a means of heightening *their* understanding, rather than getting caught up in answering and responding.

Application

As a means of identifying that which gets in the way of being person-centred:

Any training course in counselling/therapy/inter-personal skill, art therapy; any course where communicating is important (nurses. occupational therapists, teachers, youth workers, social workers, management etc); family, therapy, support groups, staff groups, self-help groups, addiction groups, marriage guidance. In art therapy. In therapy/counselling.

SESSION FOUR
Blame/Placate/Generalise/Distract/Level
with use of art
Practice in threes:
Counsellor/Client/Observer

"Go and learn how to unlearn."
Charles Pegny. Innocence and Experience

Purpose

An exercise here to show students that they knew as very young children that the person-centred approach is helpful: in remembering a teacher they liked, they pool the qualities ascribed to the person-centred approach, whereas the teacher they didn't like had the opposite qualities. Again, the purpose that they discover for *themselves*.

To reinforce the learning about the person-centred approach, and what gets in the way, the introduction of Virginia Satir's five basic behaviours: blame, placate, generalise, distract, level. Again, through an exercise, students can identify which of these behaviours is most familiar to them and, through an art therapy exercise, they are able to link such behaviour to an earlier time in their lives.

To give an opportunity to practice listening skills as counsellor, and to be able to talk further about the material which emerged in the previous exercises as client—a double sandwich—an exercise in threes: client talks, counsellor paraphrases, observer gives feedback to counsellor.

Exercise 6—Remembering a teacher you liked/disliked
'*Close your eyes. (Pause) Go back to a time when you were at school. (Pause) Remember a teacher you liked. (Pause) What were the qualities that you*

liked? *(Pause) Now remember a teacher you didn't like. (Pause) What were the behaviours of this teacher that you didn't like? (Pause).*

Students then shared the qualities of the liked teacher: 'she had time for me, she listened to me, she was caring, I trusted her, she let me be me'—And the one you didn't like?: 'she was critical, patronising, she didn't listen, she dominated, she was impatient, I couldn't speak up for myself, she didn't hear, she pretended to be saintly and was cruel.'

I suggest they hardly need to read up about the person-centred approach, as if it were a new concept: they all knew, as children, what behaviours were helpful, healthy—to be heard, accepted by someone real, honest; and those which were unhelpful—to be criticised, put down, not respected by someone they could not trust. It seems we are born knowing this. Now we need to re-connect with this wisdom, which we've sacrificed for conditional love.

It was far easier for students to remember the disliked, unhelpful teacher—far fewer memories of a helpful one. Such is the climate in which we grow up, by which we gain our self-concept. 'I'm criticised a lot, ignored a lot. I can't be much.'

As personal development is so central to person-centred training, I offer another model by which to discover learned behaviours that may impede the person-centred way of being. I talk of Virginia Satir's five basic behaviours: blame, placate, generalise, distract, level. The first four put the focus, the responsibility, away from me; the fifth, level position, is the congruent, responsible, person-centred one.

Blame:	It's your fault.
Placate:	It'll turn out alright.
Generalise:	Everyone feels like this.
Distract:	Look! there's an aeroplane.
Level:	I think—feel—want—don't want.

*Exercise 7—Role play:
Blame/Placate/Generalise/Distract/Level*
They form two circles of six.
Each one takes on one of these five 'labels'. Then they plan an outing for half-term, each speaking from that 'label'. After a few minutes they rotate, each student continuing the 'negotiation' from another 'label'. They rotate in this way till each student has had a chance to sample each of the five positions.
Then they 'debrief' in the group: which position spoke to them most/least. How did they feel in response to others, in themselves.

Rosemary found levelling hard.

Geraldine got annoyed not to be heard from the level position.

Mary disliked placating.

Heather enjoyed distracting.

Helen wants to listen to others, and wants to be heard.

Exercise with image 5 —An image regarding Blame/Placate/Generalise/ Distract/Level
'Close your eyes—reflect on these five behaviours: blame, placate, generalise, distract, level. (Pause) Maybe you were drawn more to one. (Pause) Maybe you resisted one. (Pause) Now let a picture, a scene, float up, perhaps about such behaviours. (Pause) Maybe from an earlier time. (Pause) When you're ready, open your eyes. Portray this scene.'
Each student talks about her picture in the group.

Rosemary draws a dinner table with three plates (no people). She is sixteen years old, with father and mother. She cries. Father has returned home and blames Rosemary for the break-up of the marriage, as she was always ill, aged one. She leaves the room. Later she talks of her childhood; often being blamed. Hardly any experience of the 'level' position, which she found hard in the exercise.

Geraldine draws herself in one colour, four others in a different colour. She says: 'It's really hard becoming more level, placating less—people close to me don't like me changing.' In the exercise she found it hard being heard from the level position.

Changing, becoming more person-centred, does not necessarily mean I'll be happier, liked more. It does mean that I take more responsibility for myself.

Mary draws herself, small, with long arms, holding a large mother and father either side. Her position was to placate, make everything all right. She draws herself in mauve. A mauve circle around the three figures. She didn't like the placate position in the previous exercise. *See Fig. 7.*

Heather draws her earlier journey—she wanted to study, father says: women marry and stay at home. She needs to follow her path, to study. She leaves father off the picture. In the previous exercise she enjoyed distracting, as an avoidance of the painful blaming. Later, she gives more feedback about that journey of hers, from a blaming father, to now. She says: 'So many things you say connect with me. It is exciting, as if lots of things are coming together. Then I suddenly remember how hard it was to allow myself to come and do this course, because of the 'journey', travelling up the motorway seemed very difficult. My first remark to you as I sat down: that was a difficult journey. I am here even if I do nothing else. I realise that statement was symbolic. Being here is important at this time in my life. I get lost a little less on my way here each week.' Having been told how to journey by her father, she is finding her own road now, however difficult.

Exercise 8—Listening in threes:
Client/Counsellor/Observer
I suggest that we work in threes: Counsellor/client/observer.
Counsellor to aim at understanding fully the world of the client, and conveying this to her. Reflecting. Holding up the mirror.
Observer to observe counsellor, make relevant notes, and give feedback to her honestly.
Client may want to give feedback to her counsellor. The counsellor might find it helpful to write down the feedback she receives.
After ten minutes we rotate (five minutes 'counsellor', five minutes feed-

back), *and again after ten minutes, so that each member of the triad works from each of the three positions.*

I ask if I can join three's in turn as observer, an opportunity for me to see student's progress and to make relevant comments, teaching points. The students say yes. The student who doesn't want to contribute to the book does not accept my feedback.

About feedback: A student last year called it giving 'friendly information'. If given caringly, it feels like receiving a gift. 'Thank you for telling me this. I will reflect on what you say. I find it helpful.' A different feeling to being criticised.

Give feedback honestly, congruently. How else can I learn about myself? And receive feedback without explaining, justifying; (victim position, keeps feedback out. Shades of 'the bus was late; please don't be cross'). Allow feedback in. Receive the gift. Learn.

You can make significant discoveries from each position: Client: how it feels to be heard/not heard; Observer learns by watching another; Counsellor hears the feedback.

After the exercise, we share in the group.

Mary says: as client, 'it felt good to be listened to and heard.'

Jo says: 'I was more aware of my listening deficiencies as a result of being observer. I felt anxious as the observer. I felt I couldn't be critical. Then I was at a loss to be honest. Then I realised I'd missed a lot.' Her internal dialogue got in the way of empathic observing.

Kim says: I found it hard to hear.' Last week she said: 'Owning responsibility for not making people hear me must be the opposite side of the coin of not being listened to.'

As counsellor, she got feedback about not hearing/reflecting accurately. Worries what to say, and getting it wrong—the issue she mentioned in the first week. Perhaps all part of the same package.

29

Wendy interprets. Heather selects, leaves out some 'feeling' words (which, why?).

Jo brings up the issue of 'wider reflecting': 'You say you're feeling ill and you're smiling.'

As we learn to listen better, remember more, these wider reflections can be very fruitful:

'Last week you also talked about your father and left him off the picture.'

'I notice each time you talk of your mother, your voice drops.'

The less you think about yourself, the more you can hear/remember about the client.

It is time to monitor.

Geraldine writes: 'I had thought I had analysed myself so well and yet seeing my childhood situation visually, touched me so deeply, got me in touch so accurately with all those buried feelings. So this is art therapy!'

'During the week I had felt particularly overwhelmed with demands and pressures on me. My usual coping strategy is to reach out for a Mars bar—or the like. This time I decided to draw the way I was feeling. I was amazed at the clarity of my image on the page. A mass of different colours represented all the people who needed me! I was a huge red glowing ball—full of warmth and support for these people. Out of the ball came two black hands reaching out (for my needs). However, there was no room left on the page to meet them! The picture said everything. I felt somehow satisfied even though I couldn't change anything (right then). I didn't need the Mars bar.'

And Rosemary: 'I am struck by the power of images over mere words once again and have written a few lines to try to express this:

"My soft words are borne away as a whisper on a spring breeze
My quiet words drop from my lips and melt away like morning mist

My loud words echo around the walls of my head and deafen me
My hard words rush out to hurt, ricochet and recriminate me
But my images lie on the paper staring up at me
They know me, are my history, are me."

Kim: I found placating and distracting were easier than being level. Blaming came particularly easily—the victim in me. On the level was particularly difficult because one had to make one's wants *clearly* with no room for misinterpretation. To be unclear then gives one an easy way to *blame* others for misunderstanding you. (I recognise myself in the latter.)'

Comments

From 'client', the general feedback seems to be that the level, congruent position is hardest, least familiar, that other positions were learned in order to survive.

As counsellor, they gain feedback about the quality of their empathic listening.

Some students express sadness at discovering how the cultural model seems to be diametrically opposed to the person-centred approach. How much weeding is needed before the person-centred approach can grow. It is easy to understand, to accept the philosophy intellectually—far harder to operate. Not at all like learning a skill—much more is involved, with self-awareness the key to the door.

We have arrived at a key element of the course: self and peer assessment: the responsibility of students to give and receive feedback throughout the year, leading to the certificating.

The student does not attend only for her own learning. She has a commitment to be available to her peers, to observe them, to give them honest feedback. A shift from the more familiar pyramid where teacher does it all, the rest sit back, passive. Through self and peer assessment, then, the student can experience power-sharing, taking collective responsibility, becoming actively engaged, energised, responsible. When authority relinquishes control, power can be shared.

The person-centred way manifesting in a group.

A vital element of the course experience.

And one result; a very high level—over 95%—of attendance in groups over the years.

'A student' didn't want my feedback: I accept this and I note that this hasn't happened to me thus far. I wonder about the paradox: by saying 'no' it is possible to gain much attention. A bit of me thinks: what have I done wrong? I should get it right with everyone. Familiar stuff about taking on someone else's problem, and about the need to be perfect.

Also, we had some fun today: essential. Self-awareness can be heavy—we need to bring balance, the lighter side, to this work. I doubt if I would have survived without humour.

Application

Any training course in inter-personal skills, counselling, group dynamics.

Any group/team where communicating/negotiating is important.

For any model offering self/peer assessment.

SESSION FIVE
Acceptance

"Accept me as I am so that I may learn what I can become."

Purpose

The stepping stones to acceptance:
  (1) Theory.
  (2) Identifying the main behaviour the student finds hardest to accept in others.
  (3) Through imaging, seeing that this very behaviour is a projection, comes from some very personal experience where she learned not to like that behaviour.
  (4) An opportunity to fetch the projection back, take responsibility for it, become more accepting.

Rather than talking 'about' acceptance, being in the head, the students, by going along the stepping stones, can discover something about acceptance in a very real and personal way.

Exercise 9 : A secret
The students sit in pairs.
Each student sees if she can think of a secret about herself.
Then, without telling the secret, she tells her partner how she feels about the secret, and what she thinks her partner would think about her if she knew the secret. We share in the group:

'She would think badly of me.'

'She'd judge me.'

'I could tell her because I trust her, but noone outside the group.'

'She wouldn't want to know me.'

'Never. I could never tell.'

'I worry that someone else wouldn't accept certain behaviours of mine. Would reject me.'

We're back to 'conditional acceptance'. 'I'll love you IF'. We learn to hide those aspects of ourselves which might not be accepted out there.

So, to reach a position of acceptance I need first of all to accept and love all of me, including the dark aspects. Then, only then, can I offer acceptance to another, so that she, in turn, might be enabled to accept the 'unacceptable' in herself. If there is a behaviour of mine I feel 'secret' about, I do not accept, I will not be able to accept it in someone else. As with congruence, acceptance is not a skill to swat up. Rather, much personal awareness and responsibility is required first.

Acceptance means, that I accept you, totally, throughout our interactions, whatever behaviours you may be manifesting. The behaviour is not the person. I may not behave in this way myself. However, I accept you as someone who, for the present, does. 'Accept me as I am, so I may learn what I may become'. If you don't accept me, I need to defend myself, deny, pretend. I can't go on. I'm stuck. Only when you accept me, can I look at this behaviour, and have the possibility to know it, relinquish it, and to move on.

Exercise 10—Non-acceptance
Each student writes down a list of the kind of behaviours she'd find most difficult in others. She prioritises these behaviours.
We pool the 'top of the list' behaviours: 'violent', 'child sex abusers', 'sadistic', talking non-stop', 'dogmatic', 'get ill to control', 'critical', 'bigoted', 'racist', 'ignore you', 'cruel to children'.
Between us, we eliminate a large part of the population!

Exercise with image 6—Least acceptable behaviour
'Close your eyes. Let your mind go blank. Now recall that one behaviour you found most difficult—(Pause)—
See if you can link that behaviour in some way to your own life (Pause)—See if some scene, image emerges for you to do with this behaviour, perhaps from the past—(Pause)—When you're ready, open your eyes, and portray the

image that comes to you.'
The students talk about their image in the group:

Wendy draws herself, as a little girl, watching her nurse lock her sister up in a cupboard. She feels helpless. Her 'top hate' was violence.

Dawn draws a man kissing a girl, then crosses it out vehemently. 'When I was eleven, a friend of the family whom I liked and trusted grabbed me, kissed me, put his tongue in my mouth. I felt shocked, betrayed. I haven't spoken to him since'. Her 'top hate' was child sex abuse.

Geraldine draws herself all alone to one side of the picture—noone else there—as a little girl. Her 'behaviour' was cruelty to children—it felt cruel to her to be left alone, ignored, rejected.

Jo draws a large mouth, shouting. 'Ever since ever I've had to shout, and noone hears.' Her 'behaviour' was: people who ignore you. *See Fig. 8.*

Mary's top hate was 'people who talk non-stop'. She draws herself, small, covered by a huge fog—like cloud. Mother talking, talking. *See Fig. 9.*

'When she went on and on, I felt swamped, annihilated, I don't know who I am.' Later she shares her fear of losing herself if she listens emphatically.

Heather named 'racism'. She draws herself as child in South Africa, hearing her mother being disrespectful to the black maid, ignoring her, criticising her. And a picture of her mother being ignored, told what to do, by her father.

We project out on to others internalised issues we have not resolved in ourselves. I ignore the dark side in me, and criticise it out there. The dynamic of prejudice.

A very good clue for me, when I might be projecting in this way, is when I respond to a situation with very strong feelings. I need to ask myself: how come I'm reacting so strongly? Some of this feeling may belong appropriately out there, the rest I need to fetch back indoors, to see what it's about for *me*.

I would react very strongly to all situations involving injustice, unfairness, persecution. When I did my own work about being sent to England alone, as a child, away from Nazi Europe, away from my family, I realised that those feelings largely belonged to me, needed to be owned by me. The injustice of being sent away, unconsulted—'it's not fair!' The whole issue of being persecuted as a Jew leading to my strong feelings about oppression. Now, I believe, I am available more appropriately to such situations.

Exercise 11—Counselling practice in threes
I suggest we work in triads again; one counsellor, one client, one observer, moving around three times so that each person works from all these positions.

It is important to be specific when giving feedback. Your peer can't learn much from general comments. 'You interpreted once or twice.'—Rather: when the client said..., you said...this was an interpretation.' 'You listened most of time.'—Rather: 'At one point when...you looked away; I wonder what was going on for you. The rest of the time you seemed to be listening attentively.' Give positive and negative feedback.

I say a bit more about the counsellor: as well as reflecting words, paraphrasing, focusing on feelings:

It is helpful to reflect back in a tentative mode, using words such as: 'so it sounds as if', 'perhaps you're saying', 'maybe'—so that you're not too concrete, give the client the opportunity to adjust, be flexible.—'yes, I am cross, well, actually, a bit stronger; angry, furious'.

The message you're giving is: I'm not telling you. I'm hearing you, understand what you say, I'm by you, and you're the boss. More and more, as you leave yourself aside, your need to know best, to solve the problem, you can empathise, hear, tune into the world of the client. It's almost as if you become the client, know how it is to be the client.

You may want to reflect back body language, tone of

voice, expression. You may want to offer 'wider reflecting':
'You say you like your new job and your voice is low, your
head is bent down.'
'Each time you talk about your father you sit up and your
voice is louder.'
'A student' does not want me to give her feedback after
the exercise in threes.
We share in the group:
Geraldine gets feedback about working well as the counsellor, but doing too much. She says: 'Here I go again—back to rescuer position of my childhood—having to work really hard to be noticed.'

Mary, whose issue earlier was, that when others talk, she is lost, says: 'I try to hear too hard. I am frightened of losing myself in the other person. When I try too hard I find it difficult to get in tune with the other person.'

Helen says: 'I feel it's easier counselling some people than others. If I understand, I don't block off from listening so much because I had this problem with my father trying to tell me something as a child and him getting angry if I couldn't understand. Maybe I try to understand too hard and can't hear.'

Dawn says: 'As counsellor, it is very tempting at times to use the client as a vehicle for dealing with my own stuff. 'I know exactly what you mean and if I were you'—becomes a very strong feeling.'

Nina says: 'I felt both this week and last week that in the role of client I was not making myself clear, that I had to labour very hard to make myself understood. I have felt not heard as a child (her top hate today was harming a child; not being heard felt like harm to her. Previously she had drawn a grille through which she was trying to make herself heard). I now blame myself for not being heard.'

Heather—whose issue earlier was racism—says: 'Racial prejudice has always been a problem because of childhood in South Africa. Suddenly I made the connection today with black people being ignored—the black maid being ignored; —to: women not being heard—to: my mother not being heard, to: I was not heard (last week she wanted to study, father did not hear/allow) to: I try to hear myself but keep going deaf to: as a counsellor today, not wanting to intrude on client incorrectly to: important to hear her correctly.'

Jo—whose issue was 'people who ignore you' (as she wasn't heard—even since ever) says: 'I have disclosed to myself a paradox: that I have organised my professional life as a writer and photographer in such a way that I am offered spaces to speak/show with very little facility for a dialogue. I feel clever and exhilarated and then empty, different. In another set of spaces I am beginning to want to facilitate others. Both as speaker and listener, unfamiliar with dialogue from long ago.'

Next week is half term. I suggest the students might want to take a look at the images they've produced, see if a pattern, theme, is emerging.

We monitor.

From Rosemary: 'The course work leads me to make valuable connections for myself later on: It occurred to me on the train as I travelled up today that I have suffered a lot as a result of my mother's history, and that my children have suffered in a lesser way as a direct result of my history. My mother was spat upon in the street as a "deserted" wife, and the stigma spurred her to show the world that she was as good, or better, than a man. Consequently she craved a well-paid career for herself, and sent me to an exclusive private school that I hated. I was branded a snob by cousins and the local children but I wanted to be like them. I rebelled against the elocution lessons that I was forced to take which were designed to improve my working-class accent. So I spoke differently to my school friends, and couldn't afford their lifestyles. I was socially isolated from my local peers as I went to a posh school, and furthermore my mother pushed me out to minders from early in the morning to late in the evening, as she travelled to London each day to work. If I complained I was told that I was ungrateful, as she was 'working her fingers to the bone' for me, to give me a good education. I failed to live up to her expectations when I did not pass the 11+ exam, and felt myself to be a failure even though I passed it at thirteen, and went to a technical school which I hated. I think that I went on with my studies to University level to prove to myself and my family that I was not stupid after all. I did not enjoy the academic life, and only continue to the end in order to prove that I was not a failure. It has at last enabled me to live up to my mother's expectations, and the rest of her family, my aunts, uncles and cousins, now treat me as a person of worth, instead of an insignificant member of the family. I resent this attitude, as I am in no way a different person in the important areas of feelings, warmth and reactions to people. I am amazed that the values of society reflected in my family prize intellectual achievement above personal qualities.'

Heather writes as follows: 'Looking back over my "images" I can see a few themes emerging clearly and very quickly. To simplify—"Being told" rings many bells from my childhood and the feeling of victim resulting from this—a feeling of powerlessness and impotence and being overpowered. This is reflected and highlighted by the South African situation I grew up in, where I feel a strong identification with the "powerless" feeling of the black people. I always felt appalled as if they were not there. I can see, too, how 'rescuing" grew out of this—*helping* others who are in such a situation. I don't like the feeling of "helping" but rather being alongside.

When I came to this country the one organisation I could identify with was the Samaritans because they accept anyone for any reason. I was a Samaritan for 8 years and feel I grew so much at that stage. Looking at my second image which shows lack of contact with people as a child I can see the balance swung the other way to very busy contact, almost working too much with people.

Comments

I use an exercise for students to identify a behaviour they cannot accept in others. Then I offer an art therapy exercise when students can link that behaviour in some way to their life. They discover for themselves how a behaviour they dislike 'out there' was a behaviour that had negative associations for themselves in their past.

Again we notice the power of the spontaneous image, to make such links. A vital—yet neglected—tool in teaching. Integrating reason and intuition—both needed for wholeness.

This session (and others) shows the value of using images in training. Words, theory, get you to one level. Images get you to a deeper more personal level, enable you to become more responsible for your own behaviour, to change, to move on.

Few new skills can be genuinely incorporated without this personal level of involvement and learning.

Again they work in threes, in order to practice skills, and explore further their personal discoveries regarding acceptance. Another 'double sandwich'.

Again we see that person-centred skills cannot be learned like a language, a game, a procedure. The individual needs to backtrack, discover the origin of non-accepting attitudes, before becoming more accepting.

Today's session illustrates this process.

One aspect of teaching, which I value, is that as I teach it can happen that I learn something, become aware of something, for myself.

Today, talking about acceptance, taking myself through the exercises, I note how hard it is for me, at times, to hold the balance between accepting someone's behaviour (usually someone close to me) and being congruent—outwardly as well as inwardly—about my own feelings, my own reaction to such a behaviour.

'You teach best what you most need to learn'.

A quote I like, though I don't know its source.

I realise, in the process of writing, how much of the actual experience gets lost—questions, expressions, moments of mood, mirth, excitement, frustration, non-verbal interactions, that which does not happen. I think it is this knowledge which made me postpone the writing: it can't possibly come out as a true reflection—the person-centred mirror—especially when we come to use art therapy. It won't be perfect—my old perfectionist rearing her ugly head.

So yes, some of the experience gets lost, and yes, it won't be perfect. And yes, I write on.

Application

As before.

In work to raise self-esteem.

Settings where acceptance is important. (where not?)

Situations of impasse/conflict: to resolve.

Committees, groups with more than one side involved.

Settings where prejudice (race, age, sex. religion, etc) is an issue.

Self-awareness, consciousness—raising, support groups etc.

Family therapy.

Therapy/counselling, etc.

In art therapy.

SESSION SIX
Projection
Exercise with Image: Guy Fawkes
Half Term resumé

"Do not reproach your fellow men for a blemish that is in you."

Rashi

Purpose

To bring us back together after half term, I offer an exercise of paraphrasing in the group.

We need to make a bridge from the last session—when students discovered that external unacceptable behaviour was often to do with some part of their own history—and continue with work on projection in order to become more accepting. When we project, we're not being congruent, in touch with ourselves, person-centred. We need to own the projection.

I offer an exercise in order that students can discover how they 'off-load' strong feelings of sympathy, antipathy and avoidance onto others. The element belonging to the self needs to be recognised and fetched back where it belongs. That way we became more responsible, accepting, level, person-centred.

To include an art component, I bring an exercise where the students allow images up to do with 'Guy Fawkes'. They share. They see how they project aspects of themselves onto the theme: Guy Fawkes.

They see how calendar highlights can be used as an art exercise.

To do a half-term stock-taking, the students talk in pairs about 'what I've learned so far.' They share this in the group.

I give information about Saturday, our whole day together; time, food, structure.

Some students say they have looked at all their images during the half term break as a series—and themes emerged.

Marianne says she nearly didn't come today. And felt anxious, wanted to stay away, like a truant. She doesn't know why. Now she's glad she's here.

Exercise 12—Reflecting in the round
To get us back here after the half term break, I suggest we do a brief exercise of reflecting/paraphrasing in the group: I say something about myself—a sentence or two—to the person next to me. She reflects. Then turns to the next person and makes a short statement to her about herself. And so on, right round the group. We can know from 'client' if we were/were not heard, reflected accurately. We can observe others. Just to do it—no feedback.

We move on:

Exercise 13—Projection
'Look at the people in the room. Who do you feel most drawn to? (Pause) You do not need to say who this is at any time in the exercise. Now, close your eyes. Let an image of an animal emerge for you, to do with this person. (Pause) What quality do you associate with this animal? (Pause) Where would you put yourself, in terms of distance—how far, how near—to this animal? (Pause) When you are ready, open your eyes.
Now look about again. Is there someone here you might feel yourself threatened by?' (Pause)—then the same procedure as before.
'Now look about you once more. Who is it you notice the least?' (Pause)—followed by the same procedure.

Before we go on to the next part of the exercise—sharing in pairs—I say something about projection. We saw last week that non-acceptable behaviours 'out there' were something to do with the self. We were projecting our own stuff out onto another—if I feel strong feelings of sympathy, or antipathy, or the opposite—ignoring (not wanting to see), it is likely I am projecting. Yes, the person is that way, and I am adding something of mine, probably something unaware, unresolved, as well. It is important to fetch the projection back, own it, and allow the person to be there for herself. Someone I feel drawn to, the 'hook', may be that I'm drawn to a quality I have in me, disown, and notice in another. If I feel hostile, threatened, by someone, the hook here also may be a quality I don't like in myself, disregard, and criticise out there. Not to be aware of someone—what is the quality in them I am not aware of in me? It could be about transference—another form of projection—that a person's behaviour, quality, what they say, reminds me of aspects of a significant person in my life—i.e. a parent—to which I react.

It can happen that we form relationships based on unaware projections—looking for the father or mother we didn't have, or lost, or looking for a quality which we don't own in ourselves perhaps, in another. This can skew the relationship as the partner is carrying aspects for us. I may be drawn to someone strong. Then I can stay weak, need not integrate my strength. The partner has to be strong for me, unable to activate her weak side.

We might even vote that way. Before the last election, I asked students to think of Mrs Thatcher, and see what image came up for them. One woman had a lighthouse on a solid rock: Thatcher the dependable, the strong one. Her own mother was weak, unavailable to her. She wanted to vote for Thatcher. A student drew a despot—her father: authoritarian, critical, controlling. She wanted to vote Labour. Can we elect our government based, in part, on unaware projection?!

In counselling, it is important to be aware of any projections put onto the client, to take them back, and so be responsible for oneself, and more available to the client. On this course often I pull projections to do with teacher, authority, parent.

Geraldine says here: 'Yes, the first time I saw you I knew you wouldn't like me. Now I see I was projecting an old pattern on to you of previous tutors who didn't like me.'

Now I suggest they work in pairs, taking turns to go through the exercise, and see what was the 'hook' that drew them to each of the three people, and see if there was a projection.

We then have feedback into the group:
Jo says the 'hooks' were about her mother and father.

Heather says all three behaviours were her own which she was denying, putting out onto someone else—liking, disliking or ignoring.

Dawn was surprised by the immediate pull, and yes, she needed to fetch the qualities back to herself.

It is just such strong reactions which give us a clue that there may be a projection-component.

Again, we see the need to take responsibility for the self first.

I hand out

A LETTER FROM MY AUNT

Everything is much further away than it used to be. It is twice as far to the corner, and they added a hill, I have noticed.

I have given up running for the bus, it leaves so much faster than it used to. It seems to me that they are making steps steeper than in the old days. Have you noticed how much smaller print they use in the newspapers now?

There is no use in asking anyone to read aloud to me as everyone speaks in such a low voice that I can hardly hear them. The material in clothes is getting so skimpy, especially around the waist and hips.

Even people are changing; they are so much younger than they used to be when I was their age. On the other hand people of my own age are so much older than I am. I ran into an old friend the other day and she had aged so much that she did not even recognise me.

I got to thinking about the poor thing while I was combing my hair this morning and in doing so I glanced at my reflection and—confound it—they do not even make good mirrors like they used to do!

Exercise with image 7—Guy Fawkes
'*Close your eyes. Relax, let you mind go blank—On Saturday it is Guy Fawkes. What image comes up for you as I say 'Guy Fawkes'?*

Dawn draws a pumpkin's head. She says: 'Guy Fawkes doesn't mean much to me now. I used to go along with it.

Now I prefer Halloween's. I made the pumpkin mask; that's more creative.'

I say: 'What you've just said, Guy Fawkes doesn't mean much now, you prefer Halloween's, can you relate to it in some way, does your image symbolise something for you now?'

Dawn: 'Yes, I used to conform, do what was expected of me. Now I think for myself more, do what's right for me. And I *do* feel more creative.'

Heather draws a huge bonfire; father on one side, she on the other. She says: 'As a child, my father did the bonfire. I loved it! Such enormous, free energy! Wonderful!'

I say: 'So this father, who controlled you, and made you do what he wanted, could also produce this amazing bonfire for you.' (*Wider reflection*).

'Yes, he was controlling, and giving a good experience.'

Me: 'The bonfire is between you and your father.

Heather: 'Yes! It's about amazing energy in ME! I'm projecting it onto the bonfire! I'm like father, controlling my energy. I want to let it out, enjoy it, be free.' *See Fig. 10. (Colour)*

Marianne draws a bonfire, with her standing at some distance. She says: 'I used to be frightened of bonfires, kept my distance.'

I say: 'Does that speak to you? Keeping your distance?'

Marianne: 'Yes, there was much about which I was anxious, kept away. Less so now.'

Me: 'And today you felt anxious about coming here. Wanted to keep your distance.'

Nina draws a bonfire in very faint colours which hardly show up. She says: 'Bonfires are amazing, strong, powerful.'

I say: 'And you portray it so it's hardly visible. Is that how you show your amazing, strong, powerful side?'

Nina: 'YES!'

Kim draws a picture of Heinz tomato soup. 'It's so soothing as it goes down'—puts her hand on her throat—I reflect her movement—Today she is wearing a collar round her neck, as she fell last week and hurt her neck. It—she—needs soothing.

Geraldine draws herself looking at a bonfire through a window. 'Mother said fireworks are dangerous. I was frightened of them, watched through a window.

I say: 'Do you look at frightening issues "through a window" now?

Geraldine ponders.

Today we used 'Guy Fawkes'. Events in the calendar—Xmas, New Year, Solstices, Easter, Mother's Day, Valentine's Day—all provide 'hooks'—in image form, to release some aspect of what's around for me just now, of which I need to become aware. I project onto the image. The facilitator needs to make a bridge, to help the client see those components of the picture which are aspects of herself, made visible, via the art exercise, out there. Reclaim, own that aspect. Become aware. And so the picture gives up its message. Magical. We will focus much more on the art aspect in the next two terms.

There is some time left.

Exercise 14—In pairs: Half Term Review
The students get into pairs. And take it in turns—as we are half-way through the term—to say 'what I've gleaned, learned, discovered, so far,' about me, about the person-centred approach, about art therapy. We share in the group:

Rosemary says she is beginning to reclaim her power and ship out stuff laid on her by her parents.

Geraldine is surprised at her own material still needing attention.

Kim is asserting herself more.

Marianne is clearer about the difference between aggression and assertion.

Dawn has made big strides in self-awareness: she doesn't need to be for others endlessly, she CAN make demands for herself.

Students express surprise—perhaps this wasn't expected—at the amount of self-discoveries through this work so far.

Yes, first I need to learn to swim before I can teach someone else swimming.

Mary writes: 'I need to be strong, in the sense of not losing myself, feeling who I am, and not lost in the other person.'

Jo: 'I feel alone, not lonely, separate, yet part of a group I feel safe enough to be vulnerable in.'

Dawn: 'I have been trying to "walk up to the lions on my path"—to face the dangerous aspects—for some time. I knew I wanted to, but couldn't find out a "how to." The use of images has provided that, and yes, the lion did turn out to be just a pussycat. If I can use these techniques half as effectively in my work, then I shall feel as if I am giving my clients wonderful gifts, giving them back little pieces of themselves, or at least the opportunity to pick up little pieces of themselves.'

Rosemary writes a poem:

> I tried to use my new found skill
> at the hospital for the mentally ill.
> Empathic listening was my exercise.
> You the client I viewed through new eyes.
>
> But how difficult it turned out to be
> to listen to you without bringing in me;
> interpretations kept springing to mind
> and when I forced them away behind,
> they stayed there on the boundary
> of consciousness, wouldn't let me be.

I touched the edges of your alien world
But just as I felt I had unfurled
a small corner, you moved to another track
and my incomprehension came flooding back.
All I wanted was to be there for you
But I'll never know whether that was true.

Heather elaborates on the projection exercise: 'The zebra—free, cannot be trained, strong—the quality I'm most drawn to. Lithe cat—vital, powerful—the quality I'm threatened by. Small deer—timid, shy—the one I least notice.

I can relate to all these in myself—though I didn't want to feel like the deer, the way I felt often when younger—I don't want to notice it. I feel anxious about the power in myself—don't know what to do with it.

'"Bonfire Night" was important to me. I enjoyed it. I felt strong and happy. I could show something really positive about my father who I see was nurturing as well as dominating. The good thing is, he gave me something to fight against, although it was so difficult. Now I see this.' See Fig. 10. (Colour)

Kim: Image of Guy Fawkes: 'What came to mind to me immediately was Heinz tomato soup. I don't think that I had many fireworks nights at home, but the one or two left happy memories of warmth and fun and excitement.

I like this image as it is the first that has come to mind for many years that has warm happy associations. Liesl reflected my hand movement—I was soothing my neck which I had injured last week: the warm soup goes down to comfort.

Through the projection exercise I was able to see that my unreasonable dislike of L. was directly connected with identifying her with my mother. They both, in different ways, had to flee the Nazis and had traumatic experiences with their own mothers. Unfortunately my mother has never shared or levelled with me about her experiences and emotional journey.'

Comments

In the projection exercise the animal is introduced to separate the quality, the behaviour, from the person; the projection belongs to that behaviour/quality, not the person.

When we project, we're not being congruent, in touch with ourselves, person-centred. We need to own the projection.

Again, students can see how experiential learning leads to in-sight, how in-sight is an integral part to learning.

Today projection, and I remember a watershed in my own development: once I could stop criticising, start taking responsibility for what that criticism was about for me, fetched back the projection, then I could begin to emerge from my 'dark age'. A key issue.

Application

The projection exercise: In any setting/training to do with self-awareness.

The art therapy exercise: To reinforce self-awareness; whatever is around subconsciously can come to the surface. This is true of all exercises with art.

THE DAY
Negotiating Group Contract and Assessment Procedure: Sharing of *'Life Line'*

"Each person will make his full contribution and at the same time be willing to step aside for others."

Elizabeth Boyden Howes.
'The Choice is always yours'.

"We read from the Scriptures. But each one of us has inside him(her) his own personal scripture."

Rabbi Lionel Blue

Purpose

There are two main aims:

(a) In the morning the students form their group contract and assessment procedure. They can discover for themselves how it is to negotiate collectively in a person-centred way, a process where each student expresses her ideas and requirements, and sees to it that other group members can do the same. Each member takes responsibility for the decisions reached. Power sharing. Not, the tutor telling them what to do on the course, and what not, the tutor passing/failing them, but they taking over the process. An active energetic involvement. An important experience of the course. Also, they can learn about the group dynamic; who sits back, who takes a prominent role, who asserts herself, who lets others decide, who takes responsibility, who controls, who blames. What happens to the process when one person dominates—a valuable microcosm to take to other settings.

(b) In the afternoon, the aim is to offer a group exercise with art, whereby students can share more about themselves; they paint their 'story' and talk about it. They can see how talking about themselves with an image reaches levels mere words might not reach.

I clarify: The morning's experience is central to the course: proof of the pudding: negotiating collectively in a person-centred mode. Members take responsibility to structure their course contract and assessment procedure—procedures which, more often, are dealt with by those in authority, at the top of the hierarchical pyramid, whilst those below are not involved—simply get informed. So, today's experience about taking personal power in a more political sense is significant. The model is not about winning or losing; not about competing; rather, about listening with respect, engaging actively and reaching an acceptable outcome together.

Even if the groups of students come up with fairly similar structures, the importance is that THEY devised them, rather than someone did it for them. THEY take on the role and responsibility of, in this case, a local education authority. THEY devise the course contract, THEY assess themselves and one another, culminating in the certification procedure. THEY take responsibility for giving/or not giving/the certificate to themselves and their peers.

Exercise 15—Drawing up the Group Contract and the Assessment Procedure
The first task is the group contract: the WHAT: what have we come to do together on this course.

The students divide into three small groups—each producing a list of the 'what'. They refer to the course brochure, to remind them of some of the 'givens'.

After fifteen minutes we come together and pool and add the various points, for which there is a consensus of agreement. I act as clarifier, scribe, challenger, and to read out feedback suggestions from last year's students (the inheritance).

The energy level rises as members become engaged. One student—the one not wishing to be named—is very energetic, strong and enthusiastic in putting forward her views.

After an hour we have an agreed group contract. Out of this will emerge the personal contracts—as each student's setting, approach, creativity is unique—each student will say in what way she will fulfil the group contract. When this is to be done, and how ratified, will feature under the assessment procedure.

We have a breather and return to 'part two'—the assessment procedure—the 'HOW'. How are we showing that which we're doing, learning. When will we do so.

Again, the students start in three small groups, making a list of 'hows'. Again we gather together, pool, clarify, select, add the views of all.

The process of making decisions is slow.

Again 'a student' comes over very sure and strong in presenting her ideas. The students are split about assessment groups—how many students will read a student's portfolio, when are such groups to be formed. Students fidget. They say they are too tired to decide—shelve the decision till later in the day. We've reached saturation point.

We break for lunch—a shared lunch, with many caringly prepared dishes symbolising students' feelings about the group.

And after the lunch break:

Exercise with image 8—Life Line
I want to offer a shared exercise so that we could get to know each other more. We sit in a circle, each with a piece of paper. (I ask if I can participate—the students agree. As the purpose of the exercise is to share more of ourselves, I too want to take part. It seems appropriate. Mostly I do not take part when I need to observe, reflect, be available. Today several students commented that they appreciated my sharing).
I say: 'Draw your story, your life-line, in images, however you want.' Then—each student shares her picture, her story; we decide: anyone can facilitate, but one student by her side will do so in particular.

A very moving experience. We share much more than with mere words.

Nina and Geraldine showed a dark time, after which there was growth. The spiritual aspect featured. Mary draws her parents' grave—she draws her present relationship using the same colours. She fears closeness in case, again, there'll be the pain of loss. Heather leaves out her marriage—which failed later. Often that which is left out is significant. 'A student' shares much of her life and its traumas; I empathise and feel close.

Helen draws her 'story' in very faint pastel. I say: 'I can hardly see what you've drawn.' Helen: 'I feel very fragile, vulnerable today.' Mary says: 'I feel a warmth for the group, having shared some personal history with each other. I felt comfortable sharing a painful area for me, which is loss, and obviously a powerful area for me to look at.'

There is time left. Now students are able to de-brief the morning session, express feelings. Heather bursts out: she felt that this morning she got swept along by 'a student' and decisions were made whilst she felt cross; other students share this view. Too much unexpressed feeling was around (process) getting in the way of the shared decision making (content). Students own what happens to their power when one person is dominant—they cave in, sit on their feelings of anger and frustration, and let decisions be made in a rush, without their full attention or good will. As the feelings are expressed, the air seems to clear. Now one of the issues gets resolved, negotiated—not by one, but by the whole group: the students will all work with all group members till Spring half term, when the assessment groups will be chosen. Perhaps the other decisions might be made more easily now that process has been dealt with. This was important learning—we do seem to learn more through the difficult bits.

We end with a cup of tea.

I feel tired. Keeping back, allowing others, can take as much energy as being engaged actively, yet only by sitting back can others have the opportunity to know, do, be.

If it seems to me that, at the end of their contract-making, a crucial aspect has been left out, I might voice my perception. As the tutor, I have some responsibility as to the quality of the certificate. In terms of power-sharing, I want to own my share of power. However, my intervention would come *after* the students have had the opportunity to formulate their contract. The students can agree or disagree with me. Even with the difficult dynamic in this group, the students were able to get there for themselves in the end. Over the years I can remember just one instance when the students omitted an aspect, and then it was of secondary rather than primary relevance. This shows that, when given responsibility, people behave responsibly.

I notice that each year I can stick to my task of clarifying, of holding up the mirror, of summarising, more easily. Time was, when I had my own ideas of what should/shouldn't be included in contract-making. I might have sneaked in leading comments, manipulated, abused my power. I'm glad I can sit back more, allow, trust.

Geraldine writes: The client-centred approach to negotiating was a new and exciting concept for me.

At first I felt burdened with responsibility—it was so much easier to be told what to do. However, as the process progressed I found the participation exciting and liberating. I felt valued.

I found it particularly exhilarating to negotiate, to change our minds, to exchange ideas. To listen and be heard.'

Heather writes: 'The morning session was compelling. To work as a group *sounded* very liberal, but one member was overpowering and controlling. I tried to verbalise—couldn't. I felt dishonest, not looking at why we are divided—I am shelving it. I hope to learn to tackle it at some stage. It took me till 3.20 to speak clearly about my worries. I knew I wouldn't be happy going home with what we had appeared to agree with in the assessment procedure. I was thrilled when others spoke up and expressed their worries too; and then we all came to a negotiated decision. I feel so good about this. I no longer felt cross with 'a student'. I feel I re-activated things from the past—being told, not being considered. I have been part of a very valuable learning experience—the whole group did it in the end.

'It was like a summary for me of the whole journey. The really learning thing for me was that you, Liesl, took the risk of letting us all flounder around in the morning. I kept hoping you would rescue us. I kept hoping for a cue to give me permission to speak my mind more clearly—you didn't. I had to get there myself and this I value, as having finally spoken my thoughts, three hours later, and seeing then how this enabled all of us to then together negotiate a good contract—it was so worthwhile for me. You were even prepared to allow us to use the morning's contract for the rest of the course if necessary, if that was what we agreed to—that risk that you took has confirmed in me the value of taking risks to be congruent. Thank you.'

Mary writes: 'I feel good about being able to voice my frustration without being scared of comeback, and to be listened to. I found my place in the group'.

Marianne writes: 'I felt initial anxiety about the day. Nervous of making decisions. How exhausting it is negotiating, really trying to leave everyone OK with a decision without blaming, placating etc. Taught me a lot about exercising my own power, but not in the sense of overpowering someone else. A valuable experience.'

Liesl comments: 'Yes, it's about expressing my view, AND hearing the view of others. If only we could devise a political system based on such a premise! Such creative positive energy could be released leading the constructive decision's, healthy progress.

It's important! Perhaps we need to start in a small way,

modelling the person-centred way. As here, on this course. Perhaps some students will take their learning away; implement and model elsewhere. And thus, slowly, organically, change may occur. That is my hope.'

Kim writes: '...I found it hard to make my voice heard in our small group as 'a student' seemed very forceful and insistent but I think I was finally able to assert myself...'

Group Contact

To explore the theory

To experience—

and to apply and integrate the person-centred approach on the course and in the work setting.

The person-centred approach: Empathy, Acceptance and Congruence.

To explore the theory

To experience

and to practice, integrate and apply on the course and in the work setting the potential of images through art

and to enable the individual to release the meaning of the art image through the person-centred facilitative approach: Person-centred Art Therapy.

To allow for spontaneity

To aim for fullest participation

To produce the personal contract—

To respect confidentiality.

Assessment Procedure (completed version)

Respect confidentiality

Ratify personal contract—whole group each bring and distribute twelve copies 29th November—in two groups of six, randomly chosen.

Assessment groups of three + self, randomly chosen. Three 'yes' = certificate.

Produce portfolio of learning/evidence.

Each course member takes responsibility to work with all course members during the year, to give ongoing nurturing observations (self and peer assessment) and to give such observations in writing once per term—including Liesl.

To show understanding of the theory
experiencing
and application on the course and in the work setting of the person-centred approach and of art therapy, and of linking the two: showing understanding, experiencing and application of bringing the person-centred approach to the therapeutic use of art: Person-centred Art Therapy.

To be assessed on the criteria that each person has met the aims and objectives of her personal contract well enough.

February 17—Assessment groups chosen

May 16—Portfolio handed to first assessor

May 23—Second assessor reads portfolio

June 6—Third assessor reads portfolio

June 13—Assessment day. Certificating.

Comments

In the morning we experienced a microcosm of society:

What can happen to personal power when one person dominates. How we can give up our power; how we then feel—and, today, the value of discovering how we can reclaim our power, if we want. No need to read Fromm's 'Escape from Freedom'—how we choose totalitarian systems rather than own our own power. Far more power-full to experience this truth for ourselves, in the here and now.

That is why, in this book, I choose not to quote other well-known authors, gurus, experts to say for me what I know, why I prefer to bring evidence from people, as they are enabled to find out for themselves.

The paradox in evidence: the tougher the experience, the greater the potential for learning. In other student groups, students have reported repeatedly how surprised they are that we accomplish so much in such a short time. This, they speculate, is because the competitive element is absent: no one person has to show that she knows it all. The criteria are not about being right or wrong—rather, to co-operate creatively, looking at ideas, clarifying, discarding, agreeing, a shared contract can emerge, in a spirit of mutual respect, trust and honesty.

Learning for me: it would have been more helpful to deal with process comments from the morning's session after lunch, and then be more available to the 'Life line exercise'. I teach about unfinished process comments getting in the way of content, and here I disregard that very teaching point. When I am too closely involved, when I have no distance, it is hard, at times, for me to see the wood for the trees.

In the morning, watching 'a student' active, feelings welled up within me: I recognise a 'me' of not that many years ago, the 'me' that needed to organise, control, take over, convince others of the rightness of my view. It's important that I make this connection, don't tip my feelings of dislike of this old 'me' onto 'a student'.

A lot of my own learning during the course comes through recognising familiar—if somewhat outmoded—aspects of myself in others: the one that couldn't listen, needed to know best, solve the problem; the one that projects unawarely onto others; the one that blocked her image world, played it safe by illustrating already-known thoughts. We are the same species. I, the tutor, teaching that which, not long ago, I learned as a student. I need to keep reminding myself of this truth, to keep myself humble, accepting, respectful.

Exercises with images:

Six weeks into the course, students can see that with images they have shared more about themselves in a short time than they might reveal in other settings—families included—over much longer period of time, if ever.

Application

Group contract: any group wanting to share responsibility in decision making.
Life-line: any group wanting to know more of one another in a safe way, developing trust.

SESSION SEVEN
Books, Congruence

"What I am is good enough if I can just be it openly."

Carl Rogers

Purpose

Here the purpose is:
- a) To show my 'work' books to the students; they've discovered some of the issues to do with the person-centred approach and image-making for themselves; to read the theory, other people's work now, they'll be able to say—yes, I've found some of that out for myself. The reading will reinforce the experiential learning. The reading won't be mere 'reading about'.
- (b) To focus on the third cornerstone: congruence. About being real, open, level with oneself and with others.

To give theory.

To offer the experiential component; two exercises to discover when I'm least congruent, and to discover congruence.

Helen rings before the session, to say she is not coming, may not return. Too much is going on for her, she is afraid of the work involved for the certificate. I acknowledge her view. I mention the possibility of 'the third position': she need not leave, she need not do the certificate, and she can attend, purely for the experiencing. She liked this notion, will reflect on it and contact me.

I ask 'a student'—the student who does not want to be referred to in the book—if I can mention her anonymously when writing about the morning session of our day together, as she took such a central part in the group dynamic. She agrees. I can refer to her as 'a student' in the book.

There is feedback about the day—the relief of speaking

out denied feelings, freeing oneself to move on (though Heather beats herself up—judges herself—for doing so three hours after the event). The realisation that, in this model, I do not need to push to get my way—simply, say my view and allow others to do the same. I share my view, that power is not about control, about winners and losers, about me being right, you wrong. Power is: sitting back, and allowing others theirs. Anything else is control. To be truly powerful I have to feel pretty OK about myself. Again, personal development may well be necessary to reach that position.

I share some of my 'work' books, saying something about each. The students browse—like a mini bookshop:

This seems the appropriate time to introduce 'reading'; by now the students have experienced something of the person-centred approach, of the potential of images, for themselves. If one of them reads a Rogers book now, she might be able to say 'yes, yes, I know, I've discovered this for/on myself.' Person-centred reading! We are not saying 'no theory, no reading, only experiencing.' Rather, both are needed for real learning. And this sequence on a learning programme is my preference.

We move on to 'congruence', the third of the '3Rs'.

I clarify: Congruence is about being real, honest, level. About saying: 'I'—taking responsibility for my own statement. Basically, congruence operates in two areas: that I am congruent within myself—in touch with my inner process of thoughts, feelings, sensations. If I am not, I tend to project those unowned unaware aspects out—as we saw in the projection exercises. And secondly, that I can communicate clearly my own congruence—my feelings, thoughts, wishes etc—to others. On our day, some of us knew what we felt inside, but found it hard to be congruent, to express those feelings openly.

When I am congruent with a client, the client will be able to trust me, and, ultimately, trust herself to be congruent, real. But first of all I myself need to work on my own ability/lack of/to be real, honest, genuine. Again, the focus is on me to put my own house in order, before I can facilitate anyone else to do so. Congruence is not easy; it is not a prevalent model in our culture. Most of us are reared in a climate of 'conditional love' when we learn to deny the unacceptable aspects within ourselves for fear of rejection, disapproval. We learn not to upset others, become hypocritical and, thus, out of touch with our inner selves. Congruence entails taking risks. And to take risks I need to feel OK about myself.

In the counselling encounter. it is important to know this, take equal responsibility for myself, the counsellor, rather than focus entirely on the client and her problems.

Being congruent with the client does not mean disclosing material about my own life, but being congruent about issues that belong to the counselling relationship. I may have an unresolved issue on my mind (a bereavement, anxiety etc). I do not share that issue fully, simply say that because of it I may not be able to attend totally to the client.

Paradoxically, simply stating what's with me, may enable me to put aside, for the present, my own concern. If, repeatedly, I experience strong feelings—irritability, anxiety, boredom—when with the client, I need to say so. Again, paradoxically, this can bring about a shift. I had a client who repeated the same story week after week. Finally I said: 'You bring this 'action replay' over and over again. I'm beginning to be less engaged, perhaps slightly bored.' She burst in, how she was playing it safe, while deliberating the next risky step—and then took that step.

Being congruent means being congruent *fully*. The words may sound congruent: "I don't mind that you are late." The voice may be critical. Thus, the whole conveys a double message and leads to much confusion. Some students nod here, can identify having received such double messages since childhood.

Exercise 16—'I' statements
The students are in pairs, facing. Each says to the other, about the other, four statements beginning with:
'I notice—I imagine—I feel—I want'

We have feedback.

Marianne found 'I want' difficult. To make a demand. She had no right. Later she says: 'My mother often—always—asks me something and answers the question all in one sentence. She doesn't *allow* me to speak for myself. No wonder I find it hard to speak for myself!'

Culturally, we—especially women—are not encouraged to make a demand.

Wendy struggled with 'I imagine'. It is easier to interpret, blame, put out 'you are'—'I imagine': you are taking responsibility for your statement. When you make an 'I' statement, the other person can hear, does not feel attacked or accused, need not be defensive, go into 'fight' or 'flight', but may, in turn, respond in a level way. So, two people can truly hear each other. Some students found 'I feel' difficult and did a 'think' instead. 'I feel you need to rest'. If we were not encouraged to express feelings openly, we don't know how, we suppress. Mad bad sad glad. Feelings.

Mary says: 'Being incongruent gives me an uncomfortable feeling of falseness.'

Students discover both the difficulty and the relief of being congruent.

Exercise 17—'I'm least congruent when—'
Students are in pairs—one, client—one, counsellor—then change over—client talking about: 'I'm least congruent when...'
We have feedback in the group.

Geraldine anticipated an exercise on congruence, and worried about it in advance—stopping herself being fully in the here and now. When Marianne tried to explain, Geraldine spoke for her—rescued her— perpetuating a familiar situation for both Marianne, whose mother speaks for her, and Geraldine who developed a survival strategy of rescuing as a child.

Kim reports that when she is congruent, others can be congruent back.

Heather says: 'When I'm congruent, what will I get back from others?'

If I operate, based on the response of others, I may stop myself being congruent. I give up my power to others, make decisions with others in mind.

Wendy says: 'When I'm in a new situation, it's hard to be congruent.'

Geraldine worries if the other will be upset, and rather does a 'rescue'—old pattern—but knows if she rescues, if she's not congruent, that upsets them too. Catch 22.

Kim says her mother was manipulative; Kim didn't have a model of congruence.

Jo says: 'I'm at my least congruent when I have the most to lose. (Private world). I am at my most congruent when I know the ground rules and can choose how to act/speak. When I go solo and there's no dialogue.' (Public world).

'A student' says: 'When I am congruent I may/may not be heard.'

Being congruent means, me taking responsibility for my part. What others do with it, is their—not my—responsibility. The risk is greater with near and dear ones, when the fear of rejection is greatest. If I feel OK, I can risk being congruent.

Mary says: 'I feel very congruent in pairing with Dawn for the two exercises. Sometimes I can block myself when we are practicing; when I let go of this, I feel good and real.'

We have focused on each of the person-centred cornerstones separately; we need to notice, and have,—that there is a constant overlap, an intertwining. Acceptance, empathy, congruence, all of a piece. A plait.

Comments

Did I rescue Helen by mentioning the third position? Or was I giving her information? The thin dividing line.

When I watch some students make their own discoveries: now about listening, now about the power of an image, now about congruence, it confirms my belief in student-centred experiential learning—allowing for self-discovered knowing, the only way—in my view—to KNOW.

Students are becoming more congruent in their sharing. By now they have had the possibility to experience that this model, based on empathy, acceptance, and congruence, makes for a trusting climate wherein one can hear and accept oneself, be congruent with oneself, and thus, become more whole. The discoveries are not just for this group: how to transpose this model to other settings—plant these seeds elsewhere—is an important issue today, and throughout the course.

If I were Minister of Education, I'd introduce and implement the Four Rs—the first 'R' being 'Rogers'.

We need to begin with the children: when children can grow up in an environment in which they are listened to with respect, rather than disregarded, in which they are accepted for themselves rather than made over to the wishes of others, and when they perceive adults as genuine, rather than hypocritical, they can grow up feeling good about themselves and about others. In time, our society could contain more peace and love, less violence and anger.

I am no Minister of Education. As course tutor, if I can sow some seeds in some students to propagate this healthier way of being, I am content.

Application

Congruence: In any setting where the intention is to communicate well.

The Person-centred mode: Every kind of institution—the family, educational centres, industry, local and central government, religious bodies, legal organisations, social welfare institutions, political parties, health authorities, international establishments—could function more harmoniously and constructively when some of its members relinquish old unhelpful strategies and model a person-centred way of being.

Rogers' book *On personal power—inner strength and its revolutionary impact* is all about such transformation.

SESSION EIGHT
Sharpen up group contract.
Clarifying personal contract.
Counselling practice in the whole group

"Every good thing lies on the razor edge of danger and must be fought for."

Thornton Wilder

Purpose

To sharpen up the group contract.

To clarify issues about the personal contract, to be produced in two weeks, based on the group contract.

To practice person-centred counselling skills in the whole group: one student is 'client', half the remaining students are 'counsellors', the rest are 'observers' to give feedback. Time for counselling, time for feedback and learning points. An opportunity to watch each other, learn from each other, as against twos and threes thus far.

As the students arrive, they see the group contracts and assessment procedures of the other two student groups up on the wall. They note similarities and differences.

Marianne says: 'This is an opportunity to review our contract—so that we can get our personal contract right.' We 'brainstorm' the issues that need clarifying/including. There are two main points: to be clear how to implement and demonstrate ongoing self—and peer-assessment, and to show the understanding, the experiencing, and the application at work of the person-centred approach, and of art therapy—and linking the two.

Again we note that on the day, feelings, (process) got in the way of our completing the contract (content).

We move on now to clarify the meaning of the personal contract, which is due for completion in two weeks. They pool their ideas.

Each student will say how, in her own way, in her own setting, she will fulfil the requirements of the group contract. Thereafter she has a clear brief to proceed with assembling the writing towards her portfolio. The contract ratified by peers; again, the procedure is based on self and peer responsibility.

Helen has arrived. She says she does not want to take the certificate—the pressure is too great for her at present. She wants to attend the course. Students respond: they're glad she's back. They accept her terms of continuing on the course. Helen realises what she gains—relief from pressure—and what she loses—an involvement with assessment groups. My hope for her is that she might take some learning ahead with her for future decision making regarding a commitment.

We discover something of 'the third position': she need not do the lot, she need not leave; she can find an in-between position. She has. There is always a third position between the 'either-or' continuum', some middle ground.

Exercise 18—Counselling practice in the whole group
I suggest we practice our counselling skills in the whole group: one person being 'client', half the students 'counsellor', half 'observer'. This gives the opportunity for a richer mix of feedback, of learning, than in groups of two and three.

They agree.

Geraldine, as client, talks about the dilemma: her husband has an opportunity of working in America. She wants to stay. If she says no, he'll stay. Should she say no?

Geraldine: 'Yes. If I say "no", we'll stay.' I don't want to go. I feel so settled here.'

Nina: So just when you feel settled, the issue of leaving has come up.'

(*Nina reflects, a little off-key: the issue isn't that Geraldine has just got settled. Nina leaves out Geraldine's personal comment: I don't want to go.*)

Geraldine: 'Hm. If I say "no", we'll stay. A tiny bit of me says: maybe it would be OK to go. I switch off.'

Wendy: 'You're in a dilemma.'

Dawn: 'You don't want to think about it.'

(*Between them they reflect Geraldine's issue, Wendy needs to be more specific about the dilemma: If you say: no, your husband will do what you want, yet a little bit of you is tempted to go, feels you'll be OK. Dawn completes the reflection.*)

Geraldine: 'I don't really want to go. Events might take over.'

Jo: 'You feel out of control.' (*Here Jo interprets.*)

Geraldine: 'No, I could say "no".

Nina: 'So you don't want to take control.' (*Here Nina interprets.*)

(*A summing up is needed: Geraldine needs to hear the sequence: 'you don't want to go as you might be taken over by events. And you could say 'no'— rather than introduce the emotive word: control.*)

Kim: 'I notice you're looking up.' (*Good use of reflecting body language, giving Geraldine the opportunity to say:*)

Geraldine: 'I was thinking what I can do over there. I'm frightened to think about it. I like my work here.'

Nina: 'You enjoy your work. Are frightened to give it up.'

(*She reflects the first part. 'Frightened' is more about: 'You're frightened to think about what you might do over there'*).

Geraldine: 'It feels good to be able to say it. I won't tell my parents till it happens.'

Wendy: 'You'll cross your bridges when you come to them.'

(*Again, she generalises: Geraldine needs to hear: 'You won't tell your parents till it happens.' Also, 'it' is vague, needs specifying: 'What do you mean by 'it'?*)

Kim: 'You have a lot of fear.'

(*Interpretation. Allow the client to say what she feels.* 'How do you feel about going to America, about telling your parents?' *A wider reflection of her feelings.*)

Geraldine: (*doesn't respond to 'fear'*) 'Our son wants to go.'

Jo: 'They'll have to visit you.'

(*Problem solving—not a reflection*).

Geraldine: 'How do you mean?'

'I think my husband is looking for something there, that he could find here.'

Helen: 'You may change his thinking.'

(*Very directive, interpretive*).

'Marianne: 'Can you think of anything positive about going?'

(*She is denying the problem—she—Marianne—needs to reflect what this is about for her.*)

Geraldine: 'He lets me do what I want. I feel it's my turn to let him do what he wants. If I say "no"—he'll stay.'

Marianne: 'It's a big responsibility.'

(*Rather than reflecting: So, you think by saying 'yes' to going for once you'll do what he wants this time. If you say 'no' he'll do what you want.*)

Feedback time:

First, Geraldine:

'This person-centred approach in the group seems to induce trust so that I feel safe enough to share. I received acceptance, empathy and congruence.' She does not bring the 'negative'.

The observers give feedback:

Much accurate reflecting/paraphrasing.

Nina is given positive feedback, about reflecting well. She says: 'Did I? I didn't even notice. I was so with Geraldine.'

We see also many of the classical blocks to empathy (e.g.

interpreting, problem-solving, denying the problem). It's early days.

We change over counsellors and observers.

Kim offers to work. She talks of her husband, who has had a cancer operation in the summer...

Kim: 'I support him, putting aside my bit.' (*No-one reflects this. Very often the problem is stated in the first sentence*).

Kim: 'He's not able to bring out his feelings.

Heather: 'He's unable to share.' (*Focus on husband, away from Kim*).

...Kim: I don't know how to give him the space.

Mary: 'He's avoiding the issue (*again, focus away from Kim, not reflecting Kim's statement*).

Kim: 'He just jokes about it.'

Mary: 'You want to be able to share with him him.' (*Kim hasn't brought this*).

Kim: 'In a way I want to, in a way I don't.'

Geraldine: 'You're wary of the situation.' (*Interpretive—telling her what she feels*).

Kim: No. I feel for him.

...'A Student': You feel loss, fear. (*Interpretive—feelings not brought by Kim*).

Kim: 'It's changed everything.

...'A Student': You feel weighed down. (*Interpretive—not given by Kim*).

...Kim: 'I feel impotent—I can't help him.'

Heather: 'You feel powerless.' (*Correct reflection*).

...'A Student': You feel exhausted. (*Interpretive directive. Not given*).

Kim: 'I feel nervous and worried.' (*Says what she feels. Nobody reflects what SHE feels.*)

Dawn: 'Your family life, your future is affected'—(*an assumption, taking client away from her feelings. What's that about for Dawn.*)

We have feedback:

Kim says she feels relief at being able to share. Students

appreciate her trust in sharing. And the risk of such sharing builds more trust in the group.

Wendy says she finds working in a group new.

Dawn says she can learn a lot more from watching others in this way—even if it takes her attention away from her 'counsellor' position.

Nina: 'I arrived carrying angry feelings from work. I was amazed how quickly I could let them go, and was able to feel *right there in the moment*.

(1) I stress the importance of reflecting the client's feelings. Suggesting, guessing, interpreting them—even if the client takes them on board—means the client hasn't been able to get there for herself.

The message is: 'You need someone to tell you about you—you don't know.'—rescuing, controlling.

There is a subtle difference between interpreting, and listening *so* emphatically that you are as near as you can be, sensing the client with the client, under the client's skin.

The first, tends to be thinking, intellectualising. The second, is more intuitive knowing—with the client, and then, almost despite yourself, you might hear yourself voice a client's feeling before the client. This comes after much personal work, letting go of the need to rescue, to control, to know best, to be needed, and suchlike blocks. Only then is one free for the client.

(2) The issue of timing comes up: Helen came in too soon, not giving the client time to reflect on the previous intervention. Silence can be valuable for the client's inner process; if you can't tolerate silence, explore what it's about.

(3) The need to focus on the *client*—rather than on others in the story—this takes away the focus. She's there for herself. So: 'I notice you talk about your husband, not yourself' might lead Kim to shift focus to herself.

(4) The value of digesting feedback in order to gain insight about oneself as the counsellor. This is why supervision is vital: somewhere to explore personal issues

evoked by the client (avoiding feelings, the need to rescue, control etc.).

(5) The opportunity to be congruent from observer position; at present, students seem more able to give positive rather than negative feedback.

(6) to discover how it feels to be truly heard—or not—as client;

(7) to truly listen—or not—as counsellor. Learning on many levels.

(8) the issue of interpreting.

In the book *Facing Shame*, by Fossum and Mason, the authors describe interpreting as 'mind rape'.

A student asked another student: 'Are you feeling better now?'

(a) This was a leading question. The open-ended version might have been: 'How are you feeling now?'

(b) The student asked for her *own* benefit—needing to know the student felt OK now, before the session's end. She was rescuing herself.

A useful guideline for the counsellor is to ask herself: for whom am I making this intervention—me or the client?

If for me, then I'm unlikely to be of help to the client. If for the client, separate from me and my needs, then I'm being truly person-centred.

I hand out:

The Person-Centred Counsellor's Creed

The person-centred counsellor believes:

that every individual has the internal resources for growth;

that when a counsellor offers the core conditions of congruence, unconditional positive regard and empathy, therapeutic movement will take place;

that human nature is essentially constructive;

that human nature is essentially social;

that self-regard is a basic human need;

- that persons are motivated to seek the truth;
- that perceptions determine experience and behaviour;
- that the individual should be the primary reference point in any helping activity;
- that individuals should be related to as whole persons who are in the process of becoming;
- that persons should be treated as doing their best to grow and to preserve themselves given their current internal and external circumstances;
- that it is important to reject the pursuit of authority or control over others and to seek to share power.

From *Person-Centred Counselling in Action*
by Dave Mearns and Brian Thorne

Afterwards, Kim writes: 'I found the experience of speaking to a whole group unnerving. Sometimes several people spoke, which was confusing. Sometimes my silences were shattered. On the other hand, there was a tremendous bond in the room—I felt buoyed by people's caring empathy and non-judgmental attitude—especially welcome as it is the judgement of the outside world that I fear.

The exercise when being the counsellor was extremely useful, as I was naturally engrossed with 'the client' but aware also of the other counsellor's contributions.

Jo: 'I feel fear of being observed, yet I am happy to receive critical nurturing feedback afterwards. Just as my own observer will be honest and fair.'

Marianne: 'I think I learnt more about person-centred counselling by doing counselling/observing/feedback in the whole group than ever before. However, the thought of sharing a problem with the whole group makes me somewhat anxious.'

Comment

By week 8 it seemed about right that students might risk working in this way: from two's to three's to 'going public'. From each position—counsellor, client, observer—scope for personal learning seems paramount, the issue of working towards a qualification hardly features. Real learning.

There is, at this point, some reluctance to give, or inability to see, negative feedback.

Since the beginning of the course, students are listening more empathically. Blocks to emphatic listening are also in evidence—the road is long, the journey begun.

I see again the paradox: what a rich gift it is to notice that which *doesn't* work. Only when this has been explored, owned, understood, can we move on. The gift of the dark side. I get angry remembering my 'perfectionist' history, how only getting it right mattered, denying the gift of that which doesn't work—the very key to progress.

Application

Contract making: For groups operating collective decision making.
Counselling practice: For training groups.

Any area where real listening matters.

SESSION NINE
Attitudes re Assessment
(assessing/being assessed)

"Work on yourself and serve the world."
The motto of the Grail Knights

Purpose

To give guidelines about recording case studies.

Students are voicing anxiety about being assessed. It is important to offer a structure where they can explore the origin of these anxieties; they may not be appropriate now. I offer a guided fantasy in which they can remember old messages about achieving, and address those messages now.

To allow the possibility of relinquishing some of these old internalised beliefs, I suggest an exercise where they can metaphorically enact such discarding.

I say something about recording 'case sessions'. The purpose is to bring evidence of *you*, the counsellor; so, focus on yourself vis a vis the client. Perhaps three areas are needed: (1) I said; (2) client's response; (3) commentary, i.e. 'Here I identified—the client couldn't proceed. Here I interpreted—the client had to answer my 'guess'. Here I paraphrased well—the client felt heard, could move on.' It is equally important to record difficulties as well as strengths. You are human. It is human to err—especially whilst learning something new.

Jo asks when to start with 'casework'. I put the question back to her. Later she reports difficulty in taking responsibility for decisions—would rather be told. We talk of the difference between counselling and information giving—and the thin dividing line—often the client CAN work it out.

Joke: A counsellor is clipping his hedge; a car pulls up; the driver says: 'Could you tell me the way to Windsor please?' Counsellor: 'It seems you want to know how to get to Windsor.'

Next week students exchange personal contracts. Anxieties about self and peer assessment have been voiced. I suggest we could do a guided fantasy to help them contact old attitudes about assessment, being assessed, and possibly note which of these might be unhelpful to them now, on this course, where you are assessing yourself and others, where you are being assessed, in a spirit of 'nurturing observations' (a phrase from their contract). They want this. So: I offer something like:

Exercise 9 with image—guided fantasy re assessment
'*Close your eyes—relax—push away your thoughts—*
And now, you are entering some sort of a public building—you are in the foyer—you see a notice: 'Assessment, this way'—you follow the arrow—along a corridor—you come to a door marked 'Assessment. Waiting Room'—you go in—the room is empty except for chairs along the walls. There is a door with a notice: 'Assessment. Wait here please'—you sit down—and as you sit, waiting, you go back in time, perhaps when you were a child—to a time when you were learning. And you remember the comments people made to you—possibly parents, teachers—about your learning, your reports, exams, your achieving—(pause)—and you remember how you felt—(lengthy pause)—And now, you cross over to the other side of the room, and sit on a chair facing the one you just left—you get in touch with yourself, now—your adult self—on this course, where you are assessing your peers, and yourself, and where peers asses you—and you reflect on the belief you hold about yourself now, to do with learning, assessing, knowing—(pause)—to do with your ability now to assess others—And when you are ready, open your eyes and convey your fantasy experience to paper, however you want.'
The students draw for some ten minutes, then share, in the group—deciding that anyone can facilitate.

Rosemary—
'This is little me. My head is fuzzy. These are the messages I get: "Lazy. Not good enough. Could do better." I've got my hands over my ears. I don't know who I am. Red is anger. Then there is a gap, and this is me now, in green. Green is OK. Still some fuzziness in the head. Still believing some of that old stuff. The small red is some anger. My pose is defiant.'

Nina—
'This is me as a child. All over the place. I'm nothing. I can't hear—I'm frightened of not getting it right—so I don't get it right—a vicious circle. Me—frightened. Frightened of father's anger if I don't get it right.'
Geraldine: 'The colour looks calm.' (*rescue again*).

Wendy—
'This is me when I didn't pass—I stayed down, all my friends went up. This is grandfather—in green. He loved me. He said, just be top in one thing. This is me when I passed—father rang to check—didn't believe the result! That I could pass! This is me now—a different colour—green under my feet. I believe I CAN achieve when I apply myself. I worry if old stuff will stop me being fair now.'
Later, she says: 'I drew grandfather in green—bright new green. I see I have put green under my feet. It is from this green that my strength comes—grandfather's message. Succeed in one thing. Now I feel that spiritual matters are that one thing for me.' See Fig. 11.

Marianne—
'This is me as a child. I was left to it. Red over me. I feel small, inferior. I did have one encouraging teacher. This brown rectangle is my stumbling block. This is me now. Red all around me. Wendy: you've created your own shape around you—an interpretation (*rescue*), that's not how it is for Marianne. Jo: you're feeling solid—(*another interpreta-*

tion, not fitting Marianne.) Geraldine: the stumbling block is on its side, can't trip you up—(*another rescue. It IS a stumbling block*).

Later, Marianne says: 'I was given space, but it was not enough. It did not give me the faith in myself that I needed. I am angry with my parents for not encouraging me more—as if I wasn't worth the trouble— but I know in my heart they weren't *able* themselves.'

Heather—
'Here I am in infant school. I've done well. I'm pleased. Here I am in secondary school (change of colour) still doing well. Now father says: "it's not necessary for you to do well. 50% is OK. Stop doing so well." I reflect from her 'lifeline': father said—"women don't need education, stay at home, get married." Yes, I was very confused. I got to university without any back-up—had to do it alone.

This is me now. Pink is stronger. Green is fresher. Me: So you had to come on that plane (lifeline) to get away from father's message, to become you. 'Yes. What a harsh price to pay.' See Fig. 12.

Kim—
'This is me as a baby, surrounded by safety, love. I'm cherished and spoiled.

Here I am at five. We came to England. I don't know the language.

I feel sick—I'm frightened of failing. Here I am, being sick. Sick in my stomach. I'm never good enough. Fear of father. I needed a separate paper to do me now. Rosemary: 'Your arms are up.' 'Yes, I'm breaking out. Still tight stomach, but hopeful.'

Dawn—
'I've drawn me, now. Big, smiling. I've left out little me. The message was: could do better—even if I came top!

Now, I don't let these arrows (could do better) in. I send my arrows out: I can do whatever I want. I have the evidence.'

We share. Kim is afraid she'll perpetuate her model with her children.

I feel a huge sorrow, a Weltschmertz, looking at the pictures, at the evidence of so much un-person-centred upbringing. Alice Miller's "poisonous pedagogy". Perhaps today, again, the students have experienced for themselves how unhelpful is conditional love, leading to so many negative feelings—anger, fear, confusion, lack of confidence—getting in the way of achieving one's potential. Evidence to support the person-centred approach based on unconditional love, and the realisation, after such unhelpful conditioning, the only model we know, that the shift to being person-centred is very hard. More learning by doing. How else?

Exercise 19—Discarding unwanted messages
I bring in a wastepaper basket. I say: 'You've got in touch with beliefs, messages, internalised from long ago, which may not be helpful to you now. Think of one which may get in the way for you on this course, on the assessment procedure, and, metaphorically, throw it into the waste basket.'

They write, crumple the paper, throw it away, saying:

'I'm a failure.'

'Anxiety to succeed.'

'You don't have the right to do it your way.'

'You're not clever enough.'

'I don't try hard enough. I don't want the right things from life.'

'I am not good enough.'

'I am so anxious I wonder if I can continue.'

We agree this has been a powerful session. Later Mary says: 'I felt moved by the group sharing their images. Nina's 'jelly' feeling, Dawn's 'being me', Heather's realness, Jo's anxiety—I could identify with them all.

The exercise was important at this stage, as students focus on self and peer assessment. If they operate an old message internalised about the fear of: 'I'm not good enough'—they will find it very hard, as assessors, to be congruent, to see someone else as not good enough—project out old unresolved material.

Maybe the wastepaper exercise is symbolic: we need to throw away old rubbish in order to become what we can become—person-centred.

Kim contributes 'some random thoughts':

'Looking back on my images I realise that what seems to dominate, is fear:

Fear of displeasing.
Fear of ignorance.
Fear of unleashed anger.
Fear of doing wrong and not knowing what is right.
Fear of failing.
Fear of revealing myself wholly to my children.
Fear of my parents' control.
Fear of letting the ones I love down.
Fear of losing the bits of myself that I like and slipping back to lethargy/ignorance/misery.
Fear of changing. I might not be able to deal with what it unleashes.
Fear of losing control of all the bits around me

Why do I have to be so controlling of my environment. I have to be the giver, the decider, the organiser, the catalyst for others' success. I can glean pride and grab what is theirs for my own but simultaneously blaming them for not allowing me my own space and achievements. I don't like their 'need' of me and yet cannot let go. I cannot be me—it's too scary.

I experienced physical symptoms as L. took us through the guided fantasy. My stomach started to tense and feel

queasy. I remembered my experiences with expectations, parents' needs for children to succeed.
 My first image was of vulnerability. I was loved. Adored. Cared for.
 My second image was of starting school. Walking down corridors and losing my way. Still today I have an enormous fear of losing the way.
 My third image is me curled up at around the age of 10. Expectations/exams. I have tummy pains. Run frequently to the toilet. I vomit. This continues into my adult life. Until two years ago.
 My fourth image is separate. A new me. No tummy pains. More confident. Anxieties still concentrated, however, in the abdominal region.'

Comments

The first exercise enables students to share the directive, critical, non-person centred nature of their upbringing, and its lasting and unhelpful effects.
 Students see again how, with images, they can quickly and safely reach the source of an issue—this time, anxiety about being judged, assessed, seen lacking.
 The aim of the session is that students can begin to free themselves from such attitudes, and thus be more available when engaging in self and peer assessment now.
 The exercise for symbolic discarding is important:
 There is much evidence of the power of rituals, non-verbal enactments of a process can be therapeutically releasing, merely in the doing of it. In our rational society we tend to belittle the rituals of 'primitive' peoples. In fact, we could do well to learn, to emulate, incorporate. Again, we can see how the immediacy of the non-verbal experience can be more effective than the once-removed 'talking about'.
 The symbolic enactment may not yet get rid of the be-

haviour, but focus one's awareness on the work which needs to be done to get rid of it. A powerful non-verbal reminder. And becoming aware, the crucial step towards change.

In another student group, one woman saw a swimming pool, when she heard 'you are all entering a public building.' She had no idea what this was about, but stayed with it. Later, in the fantasy, a familiar issue came up for her; how she was always compared unfavourably to her older sister. She had finished talking about her picture. Then she said: 'I know what the swimming pool means! I am a good swimmer, my sister can't swim.'

An example how an image can sometimes know in advance! Images, dreams, intuition, don't operate chronologically; trust them! They *do* know! Paradoxically, the more you can say of an image: I don't know what it means—the more likely it contains potentially valuable information for you. When you are ready to know, you will know.

Application

This material could well be used with any group of pupils/students/trainees prior to exams, assessments, interviews etc, in order to dispel old fears about failure.

SESSION TEN
Feedback

"Each member of a group should seek out some friend whose love and ruthless honesty and insight he can trust, for only the penetrating gaze of such a friend can reveal to one the defects and obstacles which interfere with growth."

Henry Nelson Wieman—'The Growth of Religion'

Purpose

This session's purpose is to give every member in the group level feedback.

There is discussion about ratifying personal contracts:

I clarify the purpose: that peers take responsibility to check out that individual contracts cover the issues specified in the group contract. This prevents possible upset during the certificating procedure. Two years ago a student was not awarded the certificate because she had not brought any evidence from her work setting. Her one ratifier had not spotted the omission of this component on the personal contract. Since then, students have decided on more than one ratifier, to double check, to avoid loopholes. The self-peer formula means that the student herself is responsible for her contract, and the peer shares responsibility in checking the contract.

I give some practical information: another group ratified in two groups of six, and this process took well over an hour.

This group has decided to ratify as a group—12 people ratifying everyone—and they needed to complete their group contract. The students discuss. They amend their decision: they decide to read twelve personal contracts during the week. That way they will know more about one another. Next week they will ratify one another's contracts in two groups of six. They select these two groups randomly.

'Helen' says she has decided she would like to take part in the certificate—she feels more positive now. Her peers say that's fine. I have reservations about her swings of mood. I share these with Helen in the feedback exercise.

Exercise 20—Voicing paranoid fantasies to group members
Before we engage in feedback, it is important to get rid of any 'paranoid fantasies' we might hold about anyone in the group. Till these are voiced we cannot give level feedback—the harboured fantasy intervenes.

We mill around—speak out our fantasies. Nina felt I was distant to her in the early sessions. I was able to tell her that during the application procedure, when she was so persistent, ringing repeatedly, I was nervous that I might not be able to meet her needs—held myself back a bit. I felt relief at the sharing.

Dawn found the exercise difficult.

Mary was anxious at first.

Heather said it was very liberating.

Another opportunity to be level, congruent—and clear the air.

Exercise 21—Feedback: Giving/Receiving
To meet the group contract requirement about giving each other feedback this term, I suggest a feedback exercise: that we mill around, pairing off. Each person tells the other a statement of what she values, and a statement of some reservation about that person. The recipient does not explain or justify (victim position), simply thanks her partner for the feedback, and writes it down. She then gives her feedback to this partner. The two then move on to form another pair—till everyone has been with everyone else. The students agree that I join in.

In this way we can make personal contact, share in an immediate, spontaneous way, whilst at the same time recording the feedback. When we've completed the procedure, we share in the group.

Mary says it was valuable.

Rosemary was anxious at first.

Nina found it nurturing and accepting.

Wendy liked the person-to-person contact.

Heather reports that what she sees as negative about herself was given to her as positive.

Marianne is amazed how time flew.

Dawn realises that the prejudices and judgements she had made before she knew people, are 'crap'—when facing them, these views no longer belong. This is something we are capable of doing elsewhere.

We talk of the caring nature of the feedback. The voices were gentle, warm, uncritical. In this way it is possible to receive negative feedback without the need to defend. Rather, it feels like receiving a gift. I can say: thank you for telling me this. It is valuable for me to know. I will reflect on it. Learn about myself.

When a similar comment is received more than twice, there is likely to be truth here, it is worth our consideration. Some comments could be subjective projection.

We review our feedback and note our reactions—do I allow in the positive? Do I beat myself up about the negative?

Very often the positive and negative are at either end of the same continuum. With me, ' sure, enthusiastic, clear, congruent' on one end can be 'too strong, not gentle enough, patient enough' at the other. How to find the middle ground! (That third position again!)

In what other settings might you use such a model? Whatever we do here, is not just for here! How about a feedback game with your family at Xmas? There is laughter. I reflect this back. Geraldine says: 'I couldn't be so honest with my family.'

We are aware of Jo's absence. She's out of it, has missed an important session again.

Later, Mary writes: I feel warm and nurtured by the comments. I will look at the areas I need to work on—e.g. valuing myself more, being clearer.

Marianne: Learning how to make positive criticism, or being able to help people be more aware of areas in which they could improve and discover their potential, is a brave and valuable thing to do—especially for someone like me who has been conditioned to avoid confrontation.

Nina: The feedback was a warm, positive experience. People's assessment was so nurturing that I did not experience it as being anxiety-provoking at all. It was a new feeling to be criticised and yet not experience it as being judgemental. I found it an enriching new approach, one which I aim to use in other settings.

And, of the person-centred approach:

Heather: I watch a parallel of my growing going on with a girl of twelve in my class to whom I have given control of her time in the classroom. She is blossoming, talking, busy. I try the Rogers approach—it feels a bit risky at times.

Kim writes: As I was writing the personal contract I suddenly was aware that it didn't matter whether I got it right or not. If it was wrong I could just do it again. So what!

Comments

Students have discovered the difference for themselves, between criticism and nurturing feedback. Before, the issue had come up: how can I be accepting, yet give negative/positive feedback? After the experience they *know:* it's more about: I accept you. I care about you. *And* I want to comment to you about these behaviour aspects of yours in a friendly, congruent respectful way. How else are we to learn about ourselves! 'Friendly information.'

The general cultural model, based on fear of rejection, leads to hypocricy, the inability to be congruent. We say one thing, feel another. We give double messages. Words convey one thing, body, voice, another. Trust cannot thrive in such a climate. The possibility of developing a true self-image, of fostering self-esteem, is impaired.

Paradoxically, it is possible to learn the most about oneself through negative feedback, caringly given. I still remember how, as a student on a counselling course, I was told, for the first time, that I do not listen. I didn't know—that was not my own perception of me—noone had ever been so level with me before. I heard the comment, and, as a result, was able to work on my own blocks to empathic listening, and move on.

Students can—as in every session—speculate where else they might use such a model.

I look at my feedback—I still tend to look at the negative first, give it more attention than the positive. Old stuff about 9/10 not being good enough. Once I can set aside this repeat performance, I can benefit from my feedback: I can allow in and take delight in the positive feedback—the fuel to keep me going. I can learn from the negative, how, sometimes in my enthusiasm, I am perceived as judgmental. How can I hold the right tension: if I dampen down my enthusiasm, not seeming judgmental is more like 'it doesn't matter.' 'I don't care.' I don't want that. If I enthuse, my eagerness is coloured by impatience, dogmatism. I need to keep an eye on me.

Application

In any group working together: the family; family therapy; staff groups, management groups, staff/student groups, youth groups, residential setting groups etc. etc.

SESSION ELEVEN
Ratifying personal contracts

"If I am not for myself, who is for me? But if I am only for myself, what am I? And if not now, when?"

Hillel

Purpose

The purpose of this session is for students to carry out and experience another component of assessing/certificating in a person-centred way: to take responsibility for one another's personal contracts, to check that they cover the criteria indicated in the group contract, even if each student does so in her unique way, in her particular setting. The object is that when they assess each other in May, no-one can plead ignorance if material is missing, not included in a portfolio of work.

Jo asked if you showed clients the case study to be used for the portfolio; she will. We discussed this issue; needing to respect the client, level with her, ask her consent for material to be used, explain the purpose and use; the adherence to confidentiality; she may say yes, or no; she may wish her real name to be used, or a pseudonym. Being person-centred means centering on the person, the client, not doing anything behind her back, even if within the spirit of confidentiality of this course. More opportunity for congruence.

Exercise 22—Ratifying personal contracts

I asked for a copy of a personal contract to be used for the book. Nina gave me hers. The students formed their two groups of six: in one, Geraldine, Marianne, Kim, Helen, Nina and 'a student'; in the other, Jo, Heather, Dawn,

Wendy and Mary. Rosemary was ill, had 'phoned in her feedback for the group, and would receive hers by 'phone. Each student to take a turn receiving comments about her personal contract from the other group members—whether it covered the points they had listed in the group contract and, if not, what needed adding, adjusting, clarifying.

As I sat, I read Nina's contract and saw that her portfolio would not include personal development or understanding of the theory of person-centred art therapy.

I was not actively engaged, could pick up voices; to my right, I heard a very balanced imput of voices—each member, in turn, giving feedback. The sound of voices was even, caring, level, amount of participation equal. To my left, I became aware of hearing one voice predominantly louder than the rest. I had a feeling of an 'action replay' from the group contract-making day, when the same student became very dominant for a time. Now she seemed to be in charge, asking each person to say more about work. When others spoke, it was mainly in response to her questions on work. I noticed an imbalance of shared comments, and an imbalance of focus— predominantly on work. I wondered if other students could claim their power in such a model, fulfil their task of ratifying. I wondered if, in this setting, *all* the points on the contract could be addressed evenly.

Although it was in the main the student's responsibility, I, as a member of the group, had an anxiety about the quality of ratifying, and wondered if some personal contracts were left incomplete, the implications and consequences this might have later, during the assessment procedure (prophecy to be fulfilled). I was twitchy, made one or two interventions to this group about the task, and the need to watch the time. I made a rational comment about procedure. I was not congruent; did not report my twitchy feeling: how hard it was for me to sit and watch passively, as 'a student' dominated, not allowing others their space. Clearly, this scenario reactivated some old issues of mine about control and helplessness. *And* some of my twitchiness belonged to the here and now.

The group on the right had finished within the agreed time. We waited for the second group to complete. Each person said something about her contract. Some needed to alter, to add something, or to leave something out. Nina said hers had been ratified. At this point, having read it, I said in my view she had left out inclusion of personal development, of understanding the theory of the person-centred approach and of art therapy, from her contract. I was at last congruent.

'A student' said angrily that in her view the contract was complete, that I was sabotaging the group's work, I was being destructive.

Kim said she was angry.

I explained—again—the purpose of the personal contract; to say what and how the person would cover the requirements of the group contract. I refer to their assessment procedure: 'The assessment is based on the criteria that each person meets the aims and objectives of their personal contract.'

Kim, Geraldine and Helen said they would revise their contracts—though ratified.

Then 'a student' again called me destructive, sabotaging. Some of 'her' group closed ranks. Justified. Blamed. Rallied round 'a student'.

Only Marianne said she had voiced her understanding and reservations of the personal contract, but had not been heard. (In a system where one person dominates, it is very hard to be assertive, to be heard).

Jo says that the whole group now needs to take responsibility to get beyond the impasse. She suggests that next week each student brings copies of her amended personal contract, to distribute to course members for their views. This was agreed.

The session was nearly over. We still needed to decide on

the numbers of assessors—left over from the contract-making day. I was aware that the 'process' comments were incomplete, as we turned to 'content.'

Mary wanted to know the role of the moderator as regards assessment: I reiterated: Her task is to check out with students how they had arrived at their contract and assessment procedures, to ensure that the certificating process was done responsibly enough for West Sussex Education Authority to certificate the course. She had no say in their individual certificating, by then completed.

Geraldine also needed to know, as it would have relevance on the size of assessment groups—to choose the size of the groups of sufficient 'clout'.

The students decided on groups of four assessors—self and three others. Then I asked, what constitutes a certificate—how many saying: 'good enough.' It was agreed, three out of four 'good enough' was a 'pass'.

There was some feedback to the ratifying procedure which they had experienced. 'Helpful'. 'Nurturing'. 'I was anxious at first, then enjoyed it.' All this from the group who had negotiated in a shared way. 'A student' again said I was destructive and sabotaging. I reflected that she had said this three times. Time was up. I said we needed to end, even though I'm aware we were not 'finished' by any means, not with content nor process.

Mary writes: 'I was anxious about ratifying, what feedback would I give and get. It came naturally and I was pleased with the feedback I got and the way it was given to me—not attacking. I made valuable contribution to others.' Mary was part of the 'person-centred' group.

Jo writes: '...In the writing up of my own contract I experienced pleasure at the fact that I have grasped what commitment is expected of me, having transformed my fears of being assessed...The session commenced with breaking into the agreed two ratification groups and our group...soon settled to an amicable discussion of points of clarity, omissions and additions. It felt intimate, helpful, constructively critical...

...The two groups then re-convened...When the reporting got to Nina...Liesl commented that she had just read Nina's contract...and she felt that as it stood the contract would not be passed...Several key phrases from the group contract appeared to be missing...Nina and other members of her group expressed some amazement at this, then anger...'a student' in particular made some particularly hostile evaluative comments... including terms like "sabotage" and "threatening". The sub group expressed great solidarity with her and seemed to be caught up in protecting their decision rather than attempting to listen to what I took to be constructive criticism...Marianne finally spoke and said that she had pointed out that there had been some points missing from most of the contracts. She felt this should have been stressed but had not felt heard, in the end backing down into silence...

...I perceived a reticence on the part of people to stop blaming and take stock of the situation...

...On reflection I see that I have shifted drastically in the last three weeks. In the criticism of others of my personal contract I felt eager to hear what people had to offer in order to strengthen and clarify my contract.

To resolve the impasse I suggested that each member of the group bring back to the next session twelve copies of their re-written contract; six for ratification by their peer group, and a copy each for the rest of us. This was agreed...

Marianne writes: '...None of us thought anything was missing from Nina's contract...how could I be right and all the others wrong...by this time I had 'given up' in a way. 'A student' was doing most of the talking and I felt she was being dismissive...I felt we were getting away from the task, when I said this 'a student' said "that's just you shooting off."...

...When we returned to the large group and Liesl pointed out what was missing from Nina's...most of our group reacted angrily...especially 'a student' who was particularly and in my view, unnecessarily abusive to Liesl. I WAS ANGRY WITH MYSELF. I *HAD* known what was required but being so unsure of myself had not been strong enough in my conviction...Personal power, personal responsibility had been lacking in me...

...I really learnt a lot about myself...What Liesl had said last week in observations, that I gave up on myself was so clearly demonstrated today...

Time and time again I tell myself to listen to myself. I know what I'm doing.'

Heather writes: '...I was in the group with Jo, Mary, Dawn, Wendy and Rosemary. I was relieved not to have to tackle 'a student's' contract which did not seem to have much to do with Carl Rogers' person-centred approach and I wondered how the other group would tackle this....In general...it was uncomfortable to watch and for me very much mirrored what had happened during our group contract day—'a student' had dominated the group and the others had allowed her to...Liesl's straightness was seen by some group members as very threatening. It does show the risks one takes in being congruent. I am beginning to trust tho' that many members of the group will learn a lot from today given time to consider.'

Comments

A fascinating experience; I sat between two mini models, microcosms of society: on my *right*, the person-centred model based on respect, on equal sharing (the *right mode!*). On my left, the model as I saw it, based on domination of one, and the ensuing hierarchy, and strategies for survival of the powerless: justify and blame, drawing together, not able to deal with the issue before them, the one congruent member not heard. It seemed to me I was MEANT to see Nina's contract, as a way of alerting, saying, this is the issue, this is what you are aiming to do with the personal contract. Having seen her contract, I needed to be congruent.

My feedback was given as helpful information, to help clarify and complete the contract. However, when the need to defend by blaming and justifying is dominant, I cannot be heard. It is too threatening. Action and responsibility might be required. And so there is collusion for the system to continue.

I remember that at the contract-making session—a similar scenario—I could sit back. The difference: today the contrast between the two groups more pronounced, more graphic. I was more aware of it. Much for me to take to my supervision!

Directive hierarchies exist because of the collusion of all—the strong wanting to control, the weak unsure of their power, and in choosing totalitarianism, giving it to the 'strong', justifying the status quo. I am amazed how many vast issues are being enacted here, in the group, on the hoof. Such as today.

Clearly, much unfinished business remains. We need to aim to complete the process next week—the last of the term—or else it will surface inappropriately later.

We see the paradox that we can learn the most through that which is difficult. We can compare the two models to situations outside the group. So many personal, family and social models get re-enacted here; sometimes I find it hard to deal with it all, to field the projections—take care of me in the moment. The tutor, too, is human.

I am aware of another issue: how to be a tutor on a student-centre course; do I sit back and give the students *all* the power? Or, as today, can I be congruent and—having read Nina's contract—share my concern? I am here too, with my share of the responsibility.

It is hard, when in the thick of it, to get the balance right.

Application

In any situation offering shared responsibility:

Self/peer ratifying (or any other mutual task) can be applied to diverse settings wanting to operate shared responsibility, to flatten the hierarchical pyramid: any student group, pupil group, task-orientated group, training group, staff team, management team, family, group therapy, family therapy, residential group, youth group, self help group, support group, etc.

SESSION TWELVE
Was-to-have been end of term games/celebration, was dealing with left-over process

"There is no crisis without a gift for you in its hands. We seek those crises because we need their gifts."

Richard Bach

Purpose

The learning of the session became:
- a) the need to be flexible within a structure—the proposed 'games' session was abandoned;
- b) the need to voice feelings, negative feelings, before being free to move on to more imput. The knowledge that if this does not happen, if the feelings are kept under, they surface again, out of context, later.
- c) more learning about the importance of being congruent, however difficult;
- d) the opportunity to discover, to take responsibility for how we respond to control (collude, give up our power, rebel, or assert ourselves);
- e) learn about the dynamic in the group. Be more aware of it.

We begin at two. 'A student' is not here.

I say it is imperative we deal with unfinished process comments—they will surface inappropriately in the future. Even if we need to delay our programme for today.

I offer to share mine—as recorded after the last session in my comments. I do. Mary asks me if some of my anxiety was about Crawley College. My fear, if the ratifying procedure was done negligently, will the course retain its certificate? Yes, perhaps another component. But also, that I, as tutor, need to take my part of the responsibility. This, I believe, I did.

Marianne says she was not heard in her group, knew they were not carrying out the procedure.

Heather says she felt as on the contract-making day, when 'a student' had taken charge. Was glad she wasn't in her group.

Geraldine and Nina justify: we did OK.

Kim thinks 'a student' pushes everything outside herself, doesn't own her issues.

We're ready to complete the ratifying in the two groups, as before. 'A student' arrives, distributes her own comments to us while the students ratify, I read this feedback: the pictures seem to be illustrations of her thoughts and interpretations (a caricature of me carrying a coffin of Carl Rogers on my back!) Whilst I'm not clear, because the comments aren't explicitly about me, the overall feeling I have is of blame and anger being hurled at me. We cannot leave this material unaddressed.

The group on my right finishes. We wait for a long time for the group on my left. Jo checks out what's with them. 'Only one to do.' We have feedback, in the whole group.

The group on the left is unresolved—two people, Kim and Marianne, did not ratify 'a student's' contract, as it was incomplete. 'A student' does not wish to alter her contract.

Jo says: 'Can you be assessed if you haven't produced a ratified contract?'

Geraldine says: 'As long as your portfolio covers the ground.' (More rescuing).

I remember our agreement, that if one group cannot agree, the issue is taken to the whole group. It is decided that the six people of the 'group to my right' will read 'a student's' contract during the holiday and bring their comments to the first session. We'll take it from there.

I bring up 'a student's' feedback and ask her for comments. She is vague—yet critical of the term's content, of last week, when not enough time was given. Jo says: 'We set ourselves one hour to ratify—that was the agreement.' Several other students challenge her—it seems since last week they became more pro-active.

The issue is brought up, that 'a student' was angry with Marianne, would refuse to be assessed by her. She is confronted some more, about rejecting Marianne, not accepting her comments on her contract.

Finally—at 3.45—'a student' comes over and hugs me. I'm perplexed: a double message. Much relief all round. There was anxiety about ending the term with negative feelings.

Dawn then brings her suggestion of an end of term tea. She goes out for cakes, I make tea. We end on a better note: an urgent need to leave us OK before the Xmas break.

Jo writes:

'The group decided to ratify each other's re-worked contracts.

...and we were told that 'a student's' personal contract had not been signed by all group members....for her part she had declined to make any alternations and seemed unable to grasp that Marianne's criticism was not an attack but a contribution towards the assessment processing going through smoothly.

...she was willing to take the consequence of deciding not to change her contract in response to sub group feedback. Liesl then reminded us that we had agreed at a previous session that if there were any problems regarding ratification that they be brought to the whole group. It was then agreed that the remaining six of us also take responsibility for reading 'a student's' contract and bring feedback to the first session after Christmas.

'A student' then spoke to her document...The first page seemed to be a series of accusations which were anything but person-centred, nurturing, empathetic or accepting. Rather they were recriminations and judgements...

...The point of a person-centred course is to encourage us to stop searching for authority figures and then blaming them, instead to find our own internal authentic and social authority, so that in turn we can model this for others.

...I felt that in the end we managed to arrive somewhere, but I felt that perhaps Liesl needed a bit of nurturing too, though she seemed strong and resolute throughout...'

Marianne writes:

'...Liesl wanted to talk about what went on last week, as did myself and others...She had felt that 'a student' was doing most of the talking and it was not a balanced process. Geraldine and Nina disagreed, they thought the group had worked well. I said I had not. I felt 'a student' was dominating the discussion but I had been unable to do anything about it and that's why I was angry with myself...

We had started on the ratifying. 'A student' arrived...

...I felt unable to ratify 'a student's' contract as it did not explicitly mention the theory aspect...'A student' refused to alter her contract...'A student' said that she hoped I wouldn't be assessing her...

Back in the big group it was agreed that failure of one person's contract to be ratified would be put into hands of whole group. Others would read 'a student's' contract again and decide next time...

On reflection:

...what's it all about? Do I remind 'a student' of somebody? Why should she react so strongly to me?...

...the beautiful part of it all is that my conditioned pattern of reacting to confrontation with withdrawal was on this occasion broken. I braved it out and came out smiling. What a lesson!'

Kim writes:

'...L. began the session: She had become anxious last

week as she sat while we were ratifying contracts. She became aware of an even hub to her right but to her left heard 'a student's' voice dominating frequently. Then her uneasiness increased at having read N's contract...
...I admired her honesty. I had never before been in a pupil-teacher relationship that was so open.
'A student' arrived at this point. She was late. (We were already preparing to do the final ratifying.)...I felt resentful.
We settled to ratify the contracts. All went well till we did 'a student's. Marianne and I refused to ratify her contract as it had no theory content. 'A student' got quite angry and said she hoped Marianne wouldn't be assessing her. I was shocked. How could someone who wanted to counsel—be accepting, non-judgemental, etc, be so vicious...
I was uncomfortable, puzzled and worried that this conflict would affect the group...
The group told 'a student' she was being unaccepting...Suddenly (it seemed to me) 'a student' got up and said she needed to hug (or receive a hug) from Liesl and then she hugged Marianne...I felt cheated. I didn't think anything had actually been resolved. I felt 'a student's' anger would surface again—it came from somewhere else. Was there some sort of transference going on here?...'A student' 'sabotaging' the group/course. Why? I didn't want to join in the 'hug'—I felt it was a ploy—phoney—a distraction. I didn't join in. Someone said "Come on, Kim." I said "I don't need to hug to show you all I like you".'

Comments

I notice that the students have contributed their lengthiest written comments after the contract-making and ratifying sessions; the two sessions with most turbulence.
We did not play 'games' as intended, could not. We had to focus on process, clear it as far as possible.
Wendy was frustrated, sees only 'exercises' as times of

learning. The other students in the main seem to have got the message; the learning from the last two weeks, though not on the timetable, was significant. Learning by experiencing.

Marianne certainly has grown through her ability to challenge. Kim too was able to assert herself.

Although group dynamics may not be part of the syllabus, it is an inevitable element and has provided us with much scope for learning—for here, and elsewhere.

The difficulties have led to more awareness, illustrated theories about power, control, blaming, justifying, colluding, person-centred negotiating, more clearly than any exercise.

During the last two sessions I am aware of my need to be understood. Some guardian angel to whisper in my ear: 'I know what you're at.' This is when I'm at risk to manipulate alliances, to leave myself less solitary. I believe I was able to note and avoid the danger on this occasion.

A little voice says: 'Why couldn't you have chosen a less problematic group for your book—we've not had any of this before; what will the reader think?' And I *know* that we gain so much from the chaos. It was *meant* to be this group, of course!

Now for a *welcome rest*!

Application

This issue of dealing with process (feelings) as well as contents (agenda/programme) is very relevant to all group-settings, from two up: committees, couples, families, management—every permutation of gathering with inter-personal issues.

SESSION TWELVE
that-might-have-been: 'Games'

"To love one's self in the right way, and to love one's neighbour, are absolutely analogous concepts."

Kierkegaard. *Works of Love*

Purpose

Usually at this juncture—end of term, Christmas-time, Chanukah, Winter Solstice—I like to introduce a more playful celebratory element, with possibilities for affirming ourselves and one another. Symbolic gifts at the season of giving.

Exercise 23—Boasts:
Participants stand in a circle.
They are invited to make a 'boast' about themselves, as if their parents were present in the room.
(I'm very tidy—punctual—I try hard etc) and then, to boast—parents nowhere to be seen: (I enjoy saying 'no'—being lazy—foolish—playful—etc).
We have feedback—often, about the difficulties of 'boasting', celebrating oneself, of internalised 'parent' messages.

Exercise 24—Love-game:
Participants are in pairs.
'a' says to 'b' (and then 'b' to 'a') a statement starting with: 'This Xmas-time I'm going to give love by...'
They change partners and say: 'This Xmas I'm going to let love in by...
They change partners and say: 'This Xmas I'll give myself love by...'
Followed by feedback.
Often, acknowledging how hard it is to be loving to oneself.

Exercise 25—Positive feedback—giving and letting in:
We sit in a circle.
Each member, in turn, receives an affirming comment about herself from all

the other members. She responds to each, saying: 'I know. I'm so glad you noticed. Thank you!'

So: 'You're a very caring person.' 'I know; I'm so glad you noticed; thank you.'

Rather than 'what! me! You can't mean it!

Often there is much embarrassment in acknowledging, allowing in, positive comments.

All these three exercises can highlight the result of upbringing in a climate of conditional love, leading to low self-esteem—a sad indictment of our prevalent culture. Also, they can put us in touch with the good, warm, joyful feelings of giving and receiving positive, non-critical comments. *Real gifts*—not to be bought in shops—perhaps representing more accurately the true meaning of the season's festivities—lost long a go.

Exercise with image 10—Gift giving:
We sit in a circle.
Each participant takes a piece of paper, writes her name in one corner, draws an outline of a container for gifts. She passes the paper to the person on her left. This person sees the name, reflects on that individual, and draws a symbolic gift (no words) of something she feels this individual might value. She passes the paper on. And so, all the way round, till it returns to the owner. She, too, might give herself a gift. Then, each participant in turn points at her gifts (no need to interpret, to know!) so that the giver can say what the gift means.

This exercise, too, makes us note how good it feels to be caring, affirming, makes us recall the flip side—how many of us were reared hearing negative, rather than positive comments about ourselves.

Little wonder, then, that by swallowing these comments we don't feel OK about ourselves.

This session, an opportunity to regain what we once knew: that we *are* OK.

A good start to the festive season.

Peace on earth and goodwill to all people, only thus.

Application

Any end-of-term, end-of-course setting.

Any setting where it is important to redress the balance of negative criticism with positive affirmations. Assertiveness training. Self-esteem workshops. Families!

Comment on whole term

We've covered a lot of ground:

The students have had the opportunity to discover for themselves their own blocks to empathic listening, to acceptance, and to congruence—the essential pre-requisite to becoming person-centred.

To begin with, their ability to listen was impaired by the need to identify, solve the problem, seek information; their own unresolved prejudices got in the way of being accepting, and old fears about rejection made congruence difficult. They could discover it is not easy to be person-centred, it takes time and much personal effort to uproot and unlearn old ways.

From client position they could discover how it feels to be listened to, accepted, and how it feels when other processes (i.e. identifying, problem solving, interpreting) occur. From observer position they could see for themselves what is helpful, what not, and they could experience giving one another caring feedback.

Their learning was reinforced step by step, with images. So they could discover the power of images and of non verbal knowing. I trust this term's evidence supports my belief that this way of learning could well be introduced on many a counselling course. On many other courses the level of learning could be enhanced with the use of the creative process, images, made visible in art-form.

They had opportunities to participate in shared decision making, to see in a very real way when this process works, when not.

On reflection, I see the difficulties of the term—particularly on the full day and the last two sessions—as a blessing. How better to illustrate and experience the two extremes on the continuum of control and shared decision-making.

We learned a great deal about the group dynamic. We

could see how all the course learning had relevant application in other settings.

A solid foundation.

And I've arrived at the end of this term, overall pleased: Remembering my feelings, before the first session, I certainly had not anticipated such a lively group! I feel excited by the ground covered—expected and unexpected—so far, and a bit apprehensive about being able to field everything that comes up in the terms ahead—perhaps I'll miss vital clues, get it wrong. Show that I'm human.

Sometimes, after a lively session, I spend much time and energy 'chewing the cud', resenting the eroding of sleep-time. The price to pay for a lively dynamic, full of potential, which requires processing. I aim to put a boundary on this process, and re-fresh myself during the break.

SPRING TERM
Bringing the Person-Centred Approach to Art Therapy

Purpose for whole term

To offer a variety of art therapy exercises so that the students:

can experience them for themselves;

can, as 'counsellor', bring the person-centred approach to working with the image;

can, over a period of weeks, note their difficulties, successes and progress;

can see how the exercises—for ones, twos, small or large groups— might be used in their diverse work settings;

can focus on assembling their portfolios and continue with self and peer assessment.

SESSION THIRTEEN
The creative process:
Theory
Messages re creativity
Exercise with image

"I regard it as possible that there may be a closer linking of our theory with developing interest in creativity in the humanities."

Carl Rogers

Purpose

1. To deal with the issue of the two students who have left. Loss/change.
2. Theory of the creative process; the difference between thinking and intuiting, censoring and letting be, left and right side of the brain.
3. To get in touch with old messages about being creative.
4. To experience an imaging exercise again based on the calendar: The New Year.
5. To share in the group, to re-connect us after the break.
6. To observe the person-centred approach with art, demonstrated by the tutor working with a student's picture—and its effect.
7. To note relevant use of today's material in other settings.

I read out Helen's letter saying she has decided to leave the course. Students comment. I myself felt early on that Helen might leave; often she was vulnerable, couldn't handle material which was surfacing for her. ' A student' had rung me to say she has decided not to continue. I had expressed regret, and accepted her decision. I hoped she might come to say goodbye to the group, for us all to have an acknowledged ending. She preferred to ring each student. (Divide and rule?) Again, we express our feelings. I say: a bit of me is sorry; we seemed to have worked through something in the last session. Also, I valued the learning offered by 'a student's' challenging position in the group. A bit of me is relieved as I may not have to manage a sometimes very difficult dynamic, field that which 'a student' brings.

It is essential to acknowledge the loss of two 'family' members, to express how we feel about this loss, to note what other feelings are evoked regarding separation from other times in our lives (one of the main themes in therapy). We need to acknowledge the changed group dynamic. Only then are we free to continue with our programme.

Jo says:

I felt confused about the purpose of 'a student's' letter from last term. I wish we could take up the issues with her present. As I feel vulnerable and fragile at the moment, I intend only to acknowledge her letter.

Kim shows a picture she drew after the 'phone call: 'a student' in the group: a big central red narrow triangle—with other group members, smaller circles, in blue and yellow.

Now we will continue without this large triangle.

I ask for helpers at the selection evenings. Prospective students come to find out about the course; I talk about the course. Applicants have the opportunity to talk to course students—just as important as talking to the tutor. I value their support greatly. More flattening of the pyramid, more power sharing. Not long ago, they were the applicants, with last year's course students to answer their questions. Now it's over to them: several people offer. The students are passing on the course torch to the prospective students.

I give the opportunity to share anything from last term or the holiday, to bridge the gap, bring us back. Heather was 'home' in South Africa; Nina's baby is due soon; Kim enjoyed an 'in the here and now' holiday.

When we are ready to move on—

The focus this term is on art therapy, in the person-centred mode. Last term we focussed on the person-centred approach. Now, a shift of focus, to art therapy, and to bring the person-centred facilitative approach to the therapeutic use of art.

To begin, something about the creative process: the 'left side, right side of the brain' model helps to clarify, illustrate. I hand out a table of left and right side characteristics from Betty Edwards' book:

Drawing on the Right Side of the Brain

A Comparison of Left-Mode and Right-Mode Characteristics

L—Mode	R—Mode
Verbal: Using words to name, describe, define.	*Nonverbal:* Awareness of things, but minimal connection with words.
Analytic: Figuring things out step-by-step and part-by-part.	*Synthetic:* Putting things together to form wholes.
Symbolic: Using a symbol to stand for something, e.g. the drawn form 👁 stands for *eye*, the + sign stands for the process of addition.	*Concrete:* Relating to things as they are, at the present moment.
Abstract: Taking out a small bit of information and using it to represent the whole thing.	*Analogic:* Seeing likenesses between things; understanding metaphoric relationships.
Temporal: Keeping track of time, sequencing one thing after another: Doing first things first, second things second, etc.	*Nontemporal:* Without a sense of time.
Rational: Drawing conclusions based on *reason* and *facts*.	*Nonrational:* Not requiring a basis of reason or facts; willingness to suspend judgment.

Digital: Using numbers as in counting.

Logical: Drawing conclusions based on logic: one thing following another in logical order—for example, a mathematical theorem or a well-stated argument.

Linear: Thinking in terms of linked ideas, one thought directly following another, often leading to convergent conclusion.

Spatial: Seeing where things are in relation to other things, and how parts go together to form a whole.

Intuitive: Making leaps of insight, often based on incomplete patterns, hunches, feelings, or visual images.

Holistic: Seeing whole things all at once; perceiving the overall patterns and structures, leading to divergent conclusions.

Through research conducted mainly at the California Institute of Technology by Roger Sperry and his students, the separate functions of the two hemispheres of the brain were revealed, showing that each hemisphere perceives reality in its own way. The mode of the left brain is verbal and analytic, right brain non-verbal, spatial. Sperry says: 'Our education system, as well as science in general, tends to neglect the non-verbal form of intellect. Modern society discriminates against the right hemisphere.'

Left side, the thinking, judgmental, cerebral, masculine principle mode. Here I am not creative. At least, I might illustrate a thought, translate it into a picture. Like a traffic signal. A cartoon.

Right side, the spontaneous, creative, intuitive, in-the-moment, non-judgemental, feminine principle mode. It is from this side, free of thoughts, that images might come, like dreams, to reveal themselves to us from the subconscious, to give up their message. We need to function with both hemispheres in order to be whole. And art therapy is one way to cross over from left side to right side, to integrate thinking and intuitive knowing. The image, when made visible as a picture, when externalised, when explored in a person-centred way, can reveal its purpose, its gift. Usually this can have the flavour of a hope or a fear, about some issue in our lives, in ourselves, which we are repressing. The image knows, and as I dialogue with it, there may be moments of 'aha', now I know—when I too see what the image is saying—not cerebral knowing, but spontaneous intuitive in-sight.

Images contain similar material, come from similar territory, as dreams. Fritz Perls says of a dream: 'It is a message of yourself to yourself, to whatever part of you is listening. The dream is possibly the most spontaneous expression of the human being, a piece of art that we chisel out of our lives.'

There is a link between the creative process and the person-centred approach, both being accepting, unconditional, spontaneous modes. To bring the two together seems most apt as a means towards self-awareness.

More about art therapy, and how to facilitate, next week—and next, and next, and next. Today, the creative process:-

We are born creative. Children fantasise; make-believe; daydream—for them this is as real as real. Small children paint carefree, large pictures. As they grow, the pictures shrink. What happens? What messages do we get about being creative?

Daydreaming, make-believe, can get judged as wasting time. Creativity—art, music—often is for the 'non-achievers', i.e. the 'non-academic'. A very negative message. Art can be taught from 'left side' of the brain: 'this is not how you draw a house', 'copy what you see perfectly'—and from the non-person-centred side: 'do it my way'. This tampers with the creative process. Gradually we put it away, conform, go for academic hurdles.

Perhaps the main purpose of the course is to reverse this model, replace with a more life-enhancing one.

I hand out a poem—about non-acceptance, of the picture, of the person. It illustrates all too well our cultural model of upbringing. The poet committed suicide aged 16.

>He always wanted to say things—
>But none understood.
>He always wanted to explain things—
>But no one cared.
>So he drew.
>Sometimes he would just draw and it
> wasn't anything. He wanted to
> carve it in stone or write it
> in the sky.
>He would lie out in the grass and
> look up in the sky and it
> would be only him and the sky
> and the things inside him that
> needed saying.
>And it was after that that he
> drew the picture.
>He kept it under his pillow and
> would let no one see it.
>It was a beautiful picture.
>And he would look at it every
> night and think about it.
>And when it was dark and his eyes
> were closed, he could still
> see it.
>And it was all of him,
>And he loved it.
>
>When he started to school he
> brought it with him.
> Not to show anyone, but just to
> have it with him, like a
> friend.
>It was funny about school
>He sat in a square, brown desk
> like all the other square
> brown desks and he thought it
> should be red, and his room
> was a square brown room, like
> all the other square, brown

rooms and it was tight and
close and stiff.
He hated to hold the pencil and
the chalk with his arm stiff
and his feet flat on the floor,
stiff, with the teacher
watching and watching.
And then he had to write numbers.
And they weren't anything.
They were tight and square.
And he hated the whole thing.
The teacher came and spoke to him.
She told him to wear a tie like
all the other boys.
He said he didn't like them and
she said it didn't matter.
After that he drew.
And he drew all yellow and it
was the way he felt about
the morning.
And it was beautiful
The teacher came and smiled at
him. "What's this?" she
said, "Why don't you draw
something like Ken's
drawing?"
Isn't that beautiful?
And it was all questions.
After that his mother bought
him a tie and he always drew
airplanes and rocket ships
like everyone else.
And he threw the old picture
away.
And when he lay looking at
the sky, it was big and blue
and all of everything, but
he wasn't anymore.
He was square inside and brown,
and his hands were stiff and he
was like everyone else.
And the thing inside that
needed saying didn't need

saying anymore.
It had stopped pushing.
It was crushed.
Stiff.
Like everyone else.

(The author has made every effort to trace the author of this poem without success)

Exercise 26: Messages re creativity

I suggest students recall the messages they received regarding creativity; they share:

Geraldine: 'I was scared of doing it wrong.'—A good stopper to the creative flow.

Kim: 'I painted to please others. And even as recently as two years ago I show my mother a picture, and she says, "that's terrible". Now I paint to please me.'

Mary: 'At school I worried if I was getting the angle right.' Judgment (left side of the brain) impeding the spontaneous process.

Rosemary: 'They said about art: it's a hobby—it won't get you anywhere.'

Marianne: 'My brother was better at art—I'd compare myself unfavourably.'—This knocks her belief in her own creative way.

Jo: 'Copying OK models, having to perform, repeating things which got praised.'

So many unhelpful messages.

If we can be less critical, more accepting of our children—more child-centred—we can learn from them and enrich ourselves. As Alice Miller writes ('For your own good'): "We will come to regard our children not as creatures to manipulate or to change, but rather as messengers from a world we once deeply knew, but which we have long since forgotten, who can reveal to us more about the true secrets of life, and also our own lives, than our parents were ever able to." A vast concept. And person-centred art therapy one of the ways towards its actualisation.

Art therapy exercises are 'hooks', aids, for us creative cripples, to re-activate our imagination, our ability to imagine more, think less. In time, we might manage to 'swim without the waterwings', it might be enough to say, 'shut your eyes—what floats up for you', or: draw/paint spontaneously—see what comes.

I suggest we do an art therapy exercise, that we debrief it, as a group—to reconnect us, after the Xmas break. It may be useful for students to be aware as they image: are they thinking, censoring, are they being spontaneous, perhaps a bit of both.

Heather remembers the first exercise of an image—hers was a crown of thorns—she edited it away—she feared it wouldn't be accepted—produced something else, something 'safer'.

I suggest there is no talking during the whole process of imaging, of portraying: words, noise, interrupt the creative process. In fact, henceforth, late-comers may have to wait outside whilst we're imaging. We will be starting each session —after any unfinished stuff, etc—with an art exercise from now on.

Exercise with image 11—New Year
'Shut your eyes—relax—breathe easy, regular breaths—clear away your thoughts, if you can—go blank—and see, without censoring, what image floats up for you, as I say: "New Year". After some minutes: 'When you are ready, gently open your eyes, and portray your image on paper, however you want.'

They draw/paint for some seven minutes.

I say—with the clock in mind—I suggest some 3-4 minutes each of sharing. I ask if first I might demonstrate/facilitate—Geraldine offers:

Geraldine: 'I don't know why—I felt happy drawing this.

These are little trees growing, and here are flowerpots with the growth not yet visible.'

Me: 'Can you associate with the trees growing, the growth in the flower pots?' (*Here I make a 'bridge', can she see anything of herself externalised in the picture?*)

Geraldine: 'It's me. Me growing. And I need rain (points) as well as the sun to grow.'

Me: 'Rain and sun?' (*I reflect—for her to say what it might mean for her.*)

Geraldine: 'Yes, I need to cry in order to grow.'

Me: Cry?

Geraldine: 'Hmm.'—(*pause*)—(*She doesn't want to pursue "crying" just now. O.K.*)

Me: 'I see you've drawn growing trees, and here, smaller pots with growth not yet showing.' (*Here I reflect two aspects of the picture—Geraldine gets there for herself.*)

'Oh yes! The trees are the free me, the pots, the cultured me—two areas of growing.'

Geraldine reports that it's the first time she's let an image come without control (the little free tree). Others work. Then she says:

'I've been looking at the picture. I've done the sun in my two favourite colours from when I was a child.'

Me: 'Your favourite colours from childhood.'

Geraldine: 'Yes, I felt happy then—as when I drew this. The happy feeling of childlike freedom. I want to reclaim some of that now.'

No judging. No interpreting. Holding up the mirror. Knowing that the client knows best. The person-centred way with art.

Again, it is important for the facilitator to start with herself: what were *her* early messages about creativity; how is it for *her* to use her imagination; how did *she* experience being facilitated with her image in a person-centred way; what did she learn? Only *then* can she begin, genuinely, to offer such an approach to others.

The beauty—one of its beauties!—of art therapy is, that art is visible, keepable. If I don't see at once, a meaning might emerge later (as with Geraldine today). Whereas words I can forget.

And, briefly:

Marianne's picture is about dancing, feeling free, happy. She loves dancing. How to transpose that feeling to other areas of her life.

Wendy draws a balloon floating, 'taking off'. She can't relate to it. Sometimes we don't see the message, aren't ready. The energetic children below needing to sleep are herself. This she recognises. *See Fig. 13.*

Heather wants New Year on her terms, not on theirs (wet paper hat—supposed to enjoy New Year), wants a New Year less busy than the old.

Often, images reveal wishes or fears not in the forefront of our awareness. Today's examples are all about wishes for a missing aspect, which have surfaced, via an image, from the unconscious. Needing to come to awareness, needing to be integrated. This integration may require further work.

We have begun! I suggest, now that they're embarking on a process of tapping into their image world, the process may not stop at 4 o'clock. They might have significant dreams, make connections away from the course.

My hope is that they look after themselves.

I say, the exercise was an example of using a calendar event as the 'hook'. Whatever is around internally will be projected onto the ensuing image, a symbolic aspect of the self made visible.

Kim asks about facilitating children of poor intellect. I give my ground rule:

Operate within the framework, the level of comprehension, the terms of reference, the vocabulary, of the person (client). Empathise with *her* world, work at *her* level. The person-centred approach can thus be effective at every level of development.

I mention the value of looking at a series of images—not just one: do similar themes reoccur, or what? As with Mary, again the fear of the 'loss of self'—comes up today.

Next week; more on art therapy: the focus on facilitating.

After this session, Geraldine contributes: 'Liesl suggested we allow an image to 'float up', and explained this was different to illustrating a thought. This idea of being 'spontaneous' is so exciting to me. I am so used to processing my thoughts and myself, that I now realise I have lost my spontaneity along the way. It is so energising to trust my real (inner) self. I was very pleased with my image. Pleased (like a little girl again), with my red and yellow sun (my favourite colours as a child).'

And Wendy got further with her image—not having understood it fully at the time—during the week. She says: 'The yellow hot air balloon, which came immediately to me, gave me much food for thought during the week. I felt it was a powerful symbol for me, saying much: a need for my own space (only one person in the basket) of calm and peace, to get in touch with higher/inner sources of strength, to be able to have a different view—overview—of what is going on around me. Ballooning does carry a 'risk'—excitement and adventure for me. It needs 'heat' to get it moving. Yellow symbolises hope for me. The jumping people below, possibly all the many members of the family that were around at Xmas—the beds with people in. And I, feeling a need to creep away and rest, sleep. In the balloon I was waving goodbye to all that!' *See Fig. 13.*

Jo: 'I drew a cane whacking down on a desk, and a blackboard, which became a window, with roses outside.

In response to reflections, I see that the cane is being held by myself—an introjected 'no'. I see the roses, but can't include them in my life. I see the empty space—feelings of despondency overcome me about Sophie's death—the empty space representing all the people I've lost, who have died. And feelings of cynicism from childhood—what's the point, people go away—my depressed self.

I felt better for having made an image, and knowing the

depth of my grief for Sophie (and myself) which I have not been able to express. *See Fig. 14.*

('She had not shared her sister Sophie's death with the group.')

The picture keeps, can continue to give up its message to us, whenever we are ready to hear.

Kim writes: 'A student' rang in the morning. She couldn't go on with the course. Her expectations were not being met. Her understanding of the principles of the person-centred approach were at odds with Liesl's. This made me very sad. I had learnt a lot from her challenging viewpoint...The devil's advocate in her/in me?...

New Year—'I knew immediately that this was a 'thinking' image as I had already thought about what to draw in the morning. However, my initial 'thinking' image became intertwined and superceded by others.

I tore a piece of sand coloured paper to depict the sand on our holiday. I then drew my family dancing with two couples on the periphery of the dance who are our friends and helped make the holiday such a joy. The green dancing figures are us and the life-giving forces. The red girl in the sand is a sand sculpture we saw on the beach. We spoke to the sculptor. I found myself worrying about the inevitable destruction of his creation. I spoke to my thirteen year old daughter about the sand sculpture—"All that time he had spent creating her only to have it destroyed," I said. My daughter remarked easily: "We made a sand-castle on holiday and that wouldn't last. It was just so much fun making it." I realised I was envious of the sand-sculptor and my daughter. The *process* was what mattered. The journey was more of a joy than the destination. I am so often going—to where?—but not *enjoying* the going.

I believe that the red is the spontaneity and vibrant processing which I would like to achieve. The grey form is the image that instantly came to my mind when I heard the words 'New Year'. This was a pelican which I saw just before we left the beach to go home. Then it was a wonderful, exciting bird to see—so unusual—but on finishing the drawing the mouth/beak looked sad and I tried to change it but it still would not smile. I could only see the pelican as a shadow over all our joys. I saw the shadow as the uncertainties connected with my husband's illness.

On finishing the imaging L. invited us to talk about what we had drawn. I couldn't take in a great deal of the other contributions. Finally I felt compelled to speak about what I had drawn. As I began L.'s voice began to question. I was phased. I asked her if she would please not speak so I could tell my story through. She complied. When I had finished she went onto the next person...I felt deflated. I would have liked her to help me move on once I had finished!

(8.7.91—I wonder if this is my strategy in life—I shut people up and then accuse them of not responding.)'

A previous course student contributed:

'To laugh is to risk appearing a fool.

To weep is to risk appearing sentimental.

To reach out for another is to risk involvement.

To expose feelings is to risk exposing one's true self.

To place your ideas, your dreams before the crowd is to risk their loss.

To love is to risk not being loved in return.

To live is to risk dying.

To hope is to risk despair.

To try is to risk failure.

But all risks must be taken, because the greatest hazard in life is to risk nothing.

The person who risks nothing, does nothing, has nothing, is nothing.

He may avoid suffering and sorrow, but he simply cannot learn, feel, change, grow, love, live.

Claimed by his certitudes he is a slave—

He has forfeited his freedom.
Only a person who risks is free.'

—and person-centred art therapy can enable such risk taking, such freeing.

Comments

In this session we need to attend to group process, to the issue of two students leaving, and to the feelings this evokes. It demonstrates, in miniature, the vast topic of loss and change. The importance of congruence is seen: when people can express feelings openly, genuinely about the two students who have left, we can move on. When such unexpressed feelings go underground, they can pop up inappropriately elsewhere, later. Helpful learning to take to other situations elsewhere. Two coping strategies, when in difficulty, are 'fight' and 'flight'. Neither leads to resolution, being strategies of avoidance. The only way forward is to face the difficulty, work through it, and move on. When someone leaves, very likely it is a form of 'flight' from something that cannot be faced at present.

In this session I re-cap about the creative process, about the difference between thinking and intuiting, between censoring and letting be, so that students can observe that process in themselves, as they experience imaging.

From theory to learning by doing—an art therapy exercise.

We see how an event in the calendar—today New Year—can be used as a focus for the image.

The theory I talked about—what can happen with images—now becomes real:

Geraldine produces an image she doesn't understand. Gradually its message is disclosed. Here, too, we see the effect of the person-centred approach with the image: reflecting back aspects of the image, letting Geraldine know—or not know. Because the image keeps, knowing may occur long after it has been created. For her, at the end of the exercise.

For Marianne it is a wish, a hope, made aware.—Most images are either hopes or fears.

Wendy shows how she got the message of her picture later in the week—the image was more powerful than words. She became aware of her own needs, which she tends to deny.

The image brings unaware material to the forefront. Material that needs to be known.

Theory into practice: the way to know.

Application

Person-centred art therapy might, at first, seem a subject merely applicable in the field of therapy.

Based on the need for both verbal and non-verbal intelligence for integrated perception, it has far wider relevance, not only for the vast range of professionals working with people, but also as a valuable resource on any teaching and training programme. This range, in a wide, general sense, applies to every session to follow. In addition, application will be listed after each session as particularly relevant to the specific material of that session.

Application—here and henceforth

Any course/training/group to do with the development of the person, where art therapy can facilitate such development. Material can be used/amended in a variety of settings working with individuals and groups.

Any setting where the facilitator holds the belief that the client knows best, that she needs to be in tune with the client's world without interpretation and judging, so that growth and integration might take place for the client.

Any course/training/group where the integration of imagination, inspiration, intuition and spontaneity, with the cerebral thinking mode is important: thus, any situation to do with the development of the person.

Any course/ training/group setting where the use of art can facilitate that integration.

Inter alia: Art therapy, the expressive therapies, social work, nursing, O.T., counselling, therapy, youth work, working with addiction, abuse, terminal illness, management, staff groups, student groups, support groups, etc. etc. etc.

This will apply to most subsequent sessions.

SESSION FOURTEEN
Guidelines for the person-centred facilitator of art therapy. Exercise with image—an animal

"I have spread my dreams under your feet. Tread softly because you tread on my dreams."

W.B. Yates

Purpose

The object of this session is:

(1) to give some historical background of art therapy;

(2) to talk about the process of imaging, and producing the image;

(3) to indicate the therapeutic potential of this process;

(4) to give guidelines to a facilitator working with art in a person—centred way;

(5) to offer an experiential art therapy exercise where:

(a) I demonstrate,

(b) the students practise as facilitator, receiving feedback from the 'observer'.

(c) There is the opportunity to experience for oneself what an image can disclose, in a very short time, how helpful the person-centred approach is for the client, how unhelpful and intrusive are interpretations, identifying, directive interventions.

(d) The opportunity to discover, the more spontaneous the image (I have no idea what it's about) the more material it is likely to disclose; an illustrated thought merely illustrates something already known.

(6) Again the need to have some theoretical imput and then, experiential discovering for oneself.

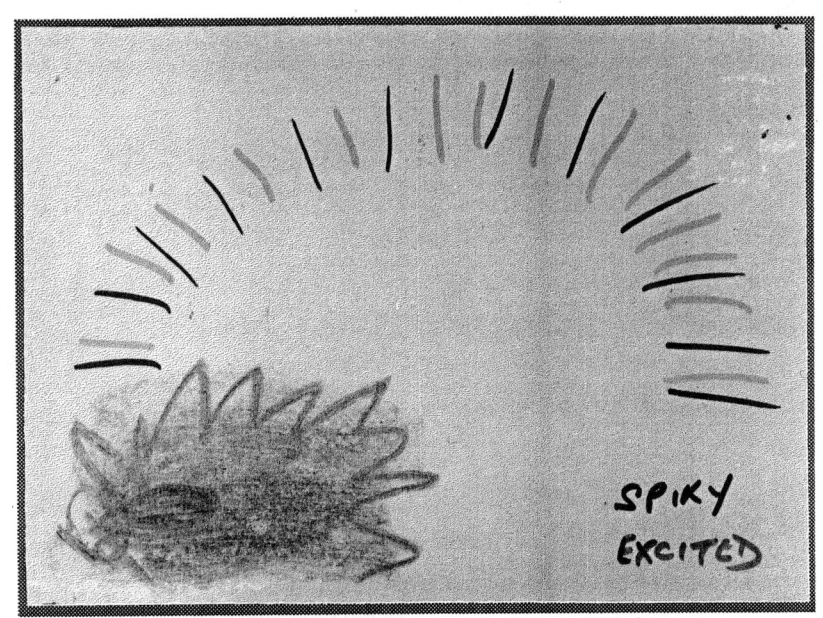

Fig. 1 (p. 6): Jo: Anxious and excited.

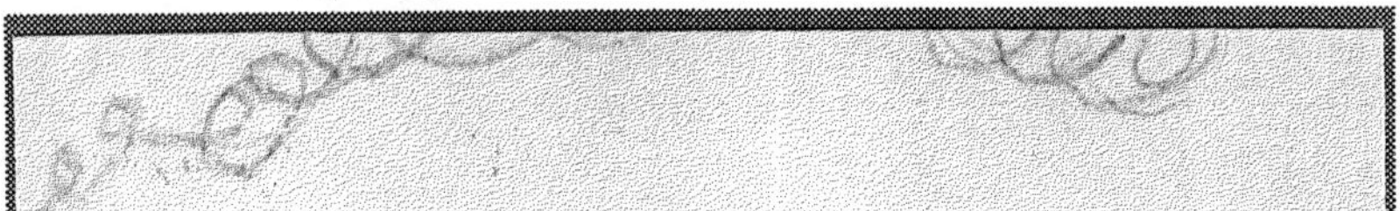

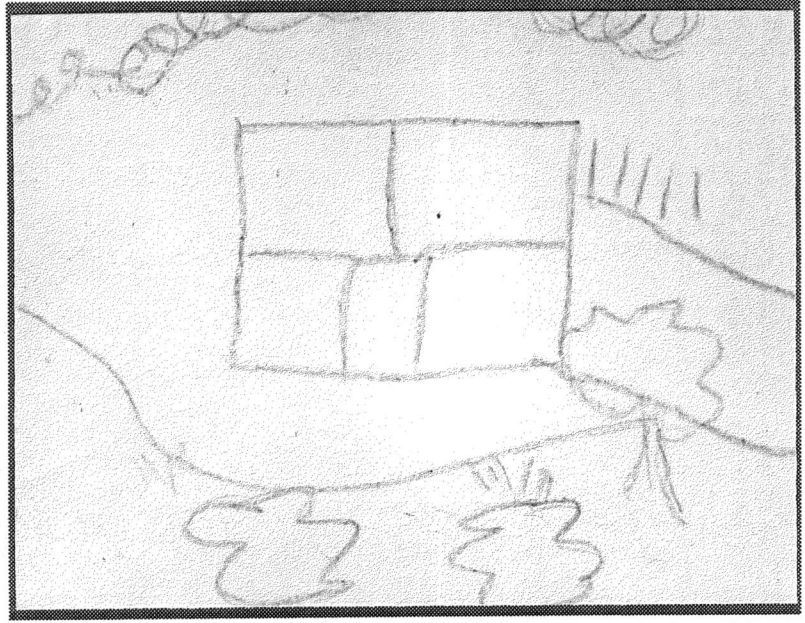

Fig. 2 (p. 15): Heather: I talk to the friendly house; people don't listen.

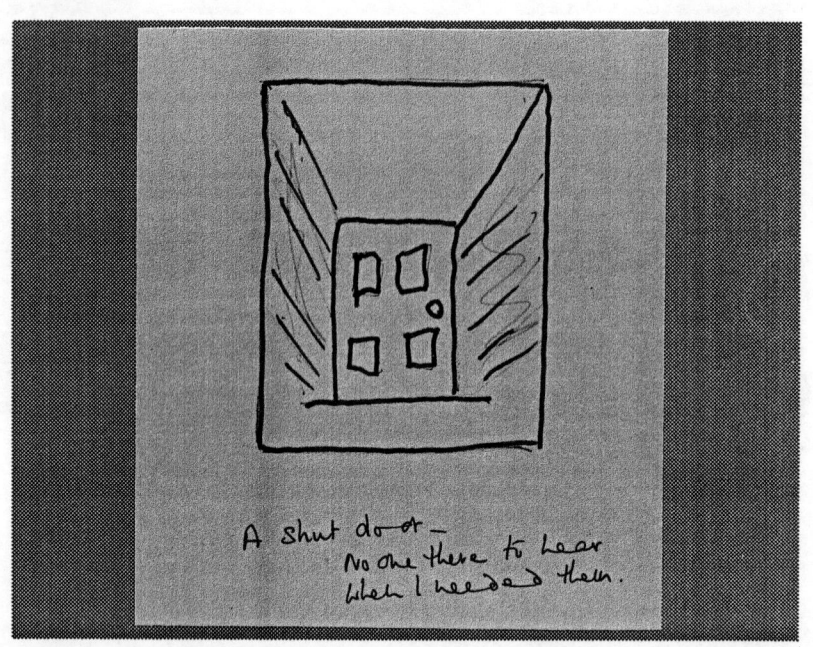

Fig. 3 (p. 15): Wendy: No-one there to hear.

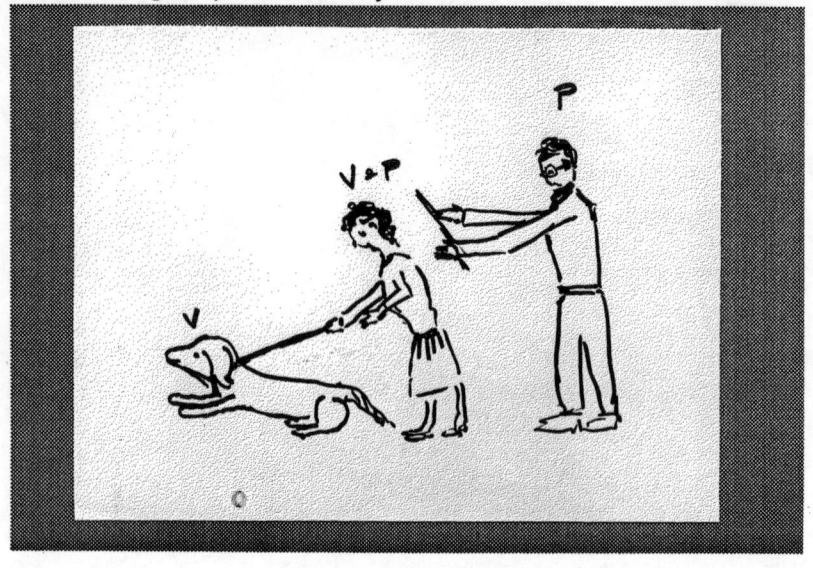

Fig. 4 (p. 22): Rosemary: 'Kick the cat' syndrome.

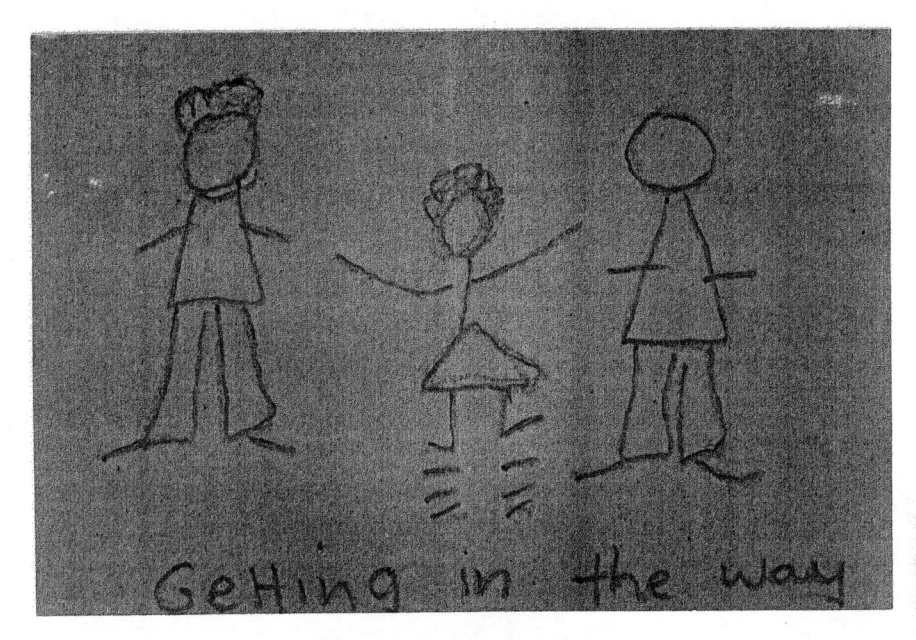

Fig. 5 (p. 23): Heather.

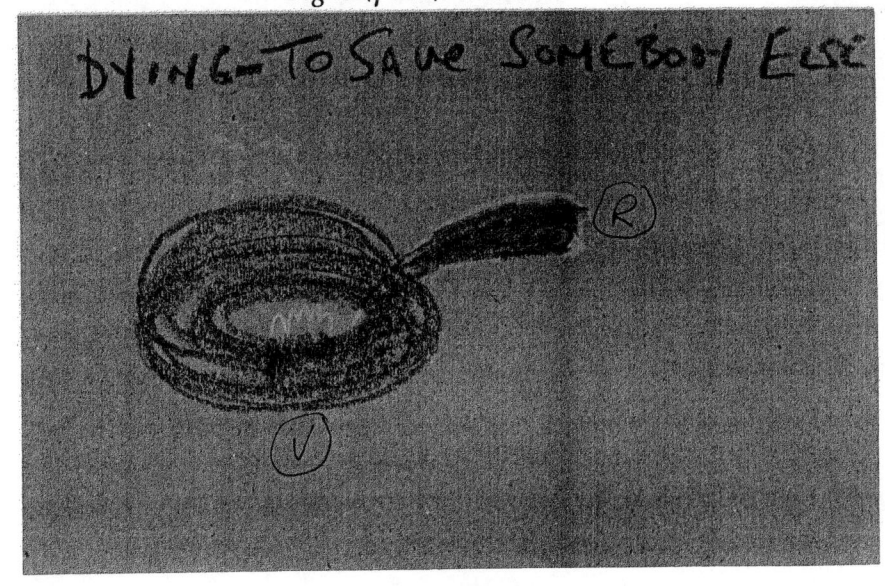

Fig. 6 (p. 23): Jo.

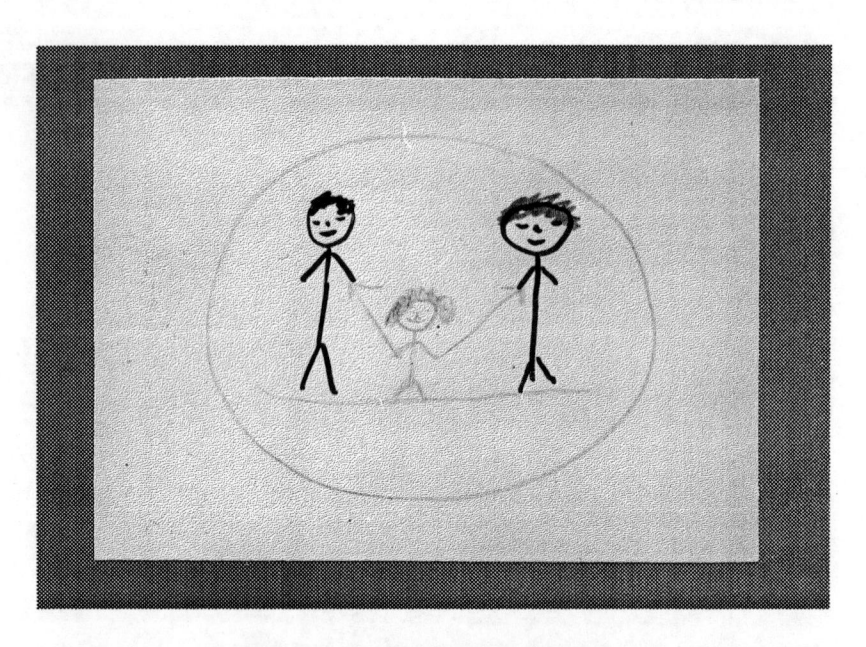

Fig. 7 (p. 28): Mary: I placate.

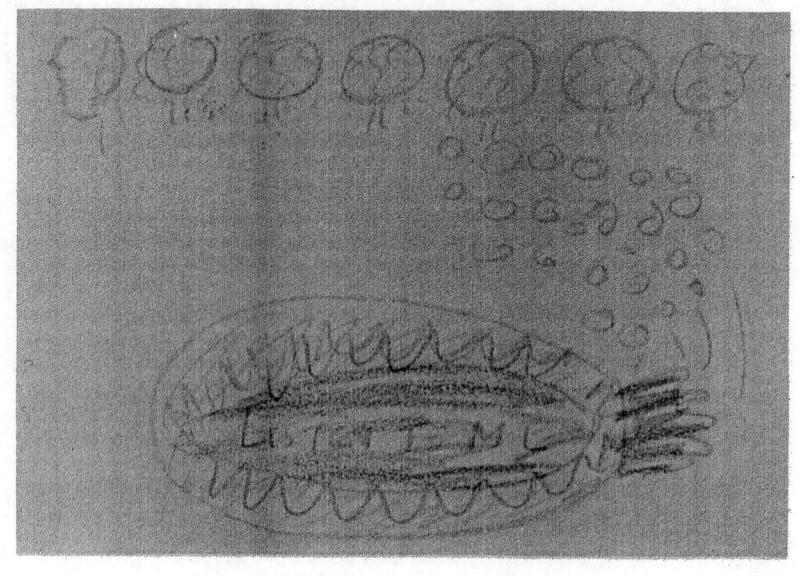

Fig. 8 (p. 35): Jo: No-one hears.

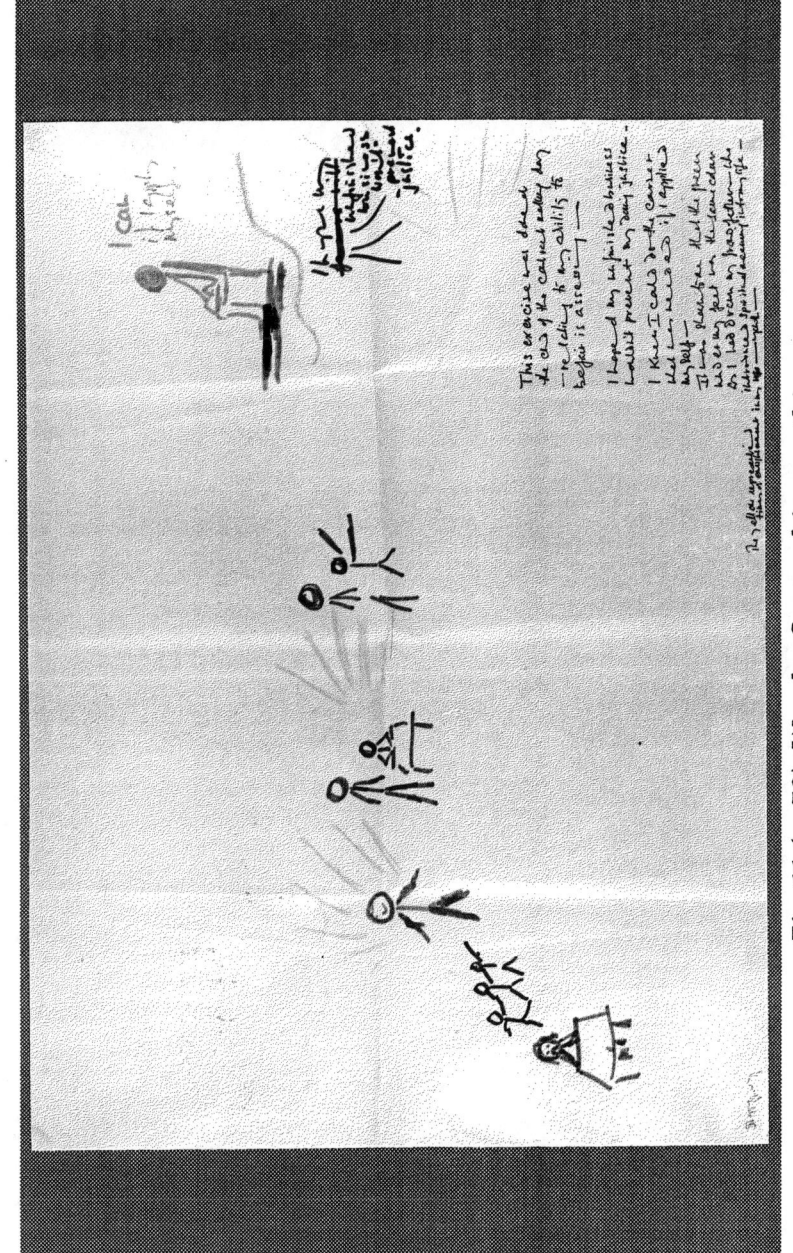

Fig. 11 (p. 79): Wendy: Succeed in one thing.

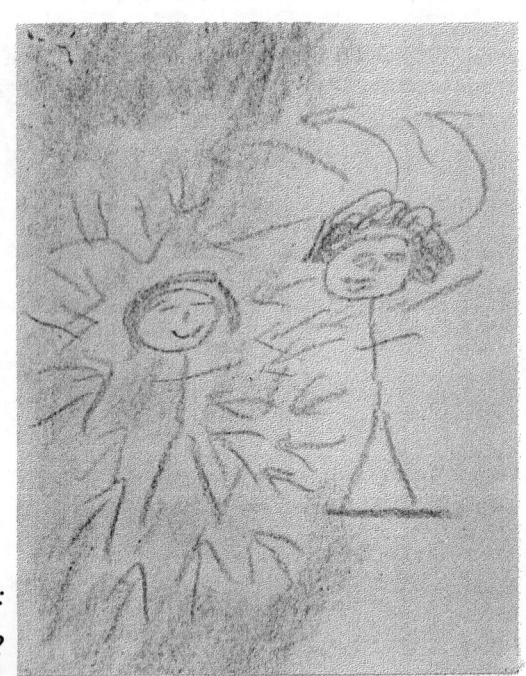

Fig. 9 (p. 35):
Mary: Who am I?

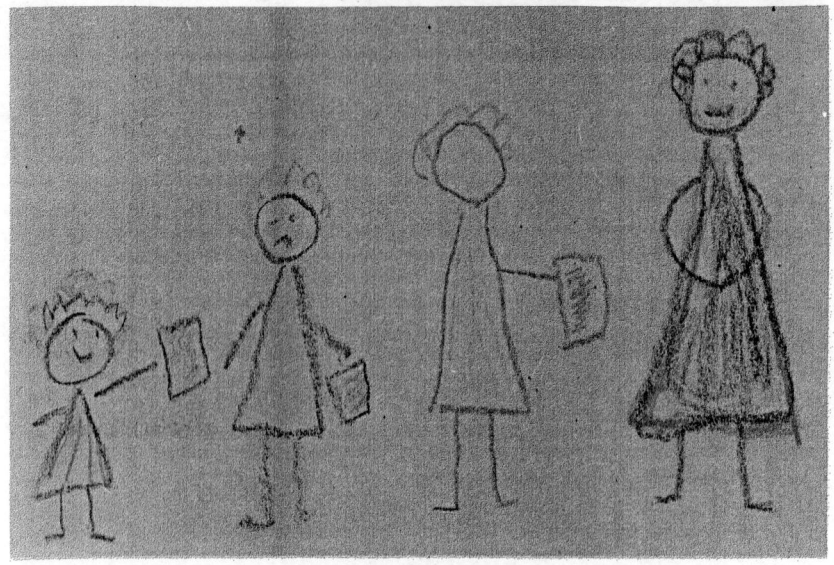

Fig. 12 (p. 80): Heather: Going it alone.

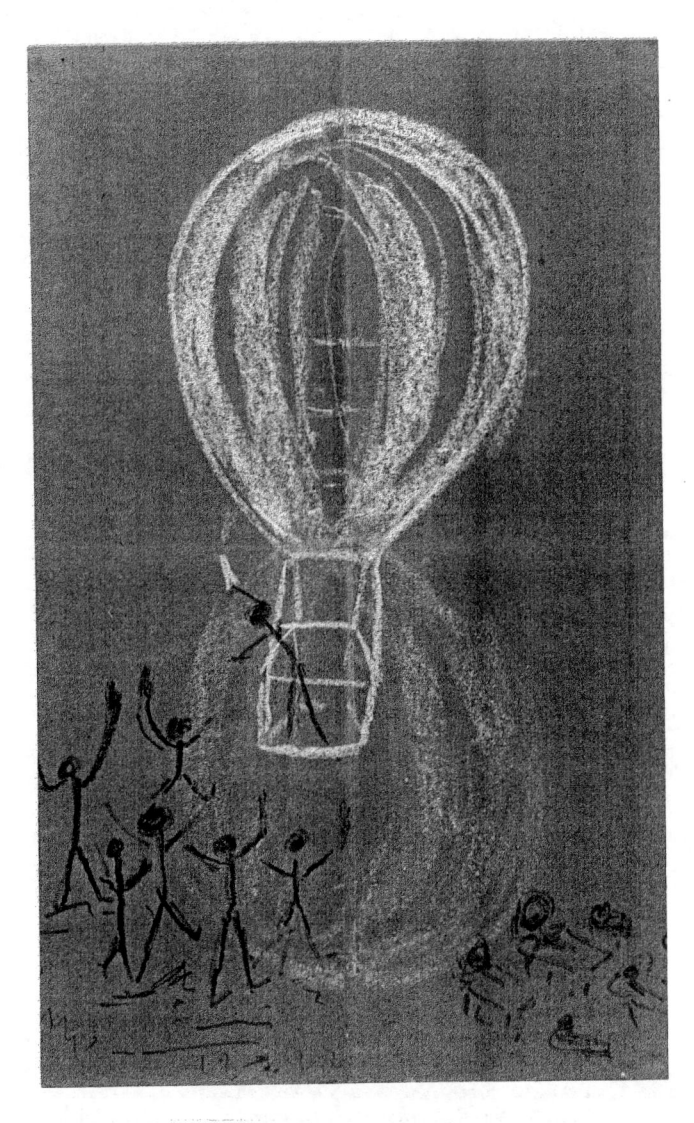

Fig. 13 (p. 123): Wendy: I need my own space.

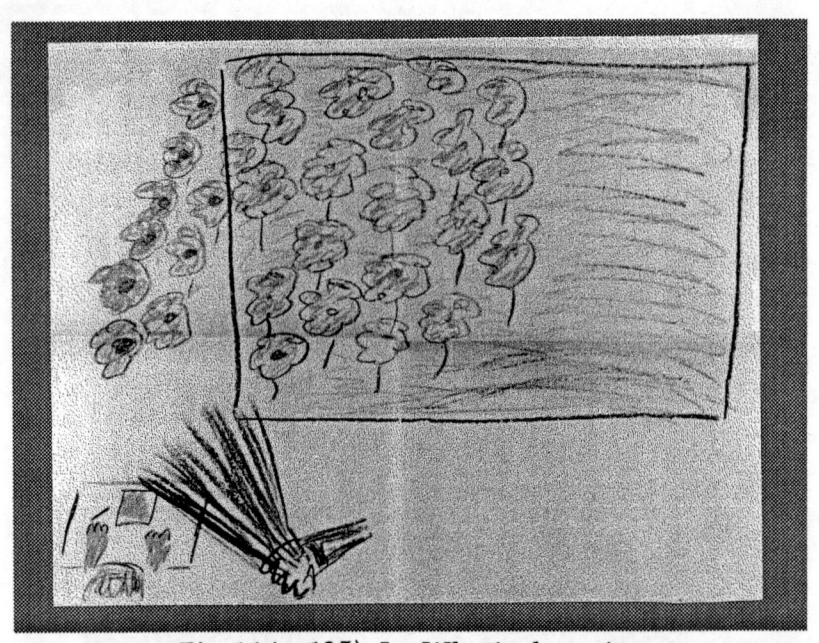

Fig. 14 (p. 125): **Jo: What's the point.**

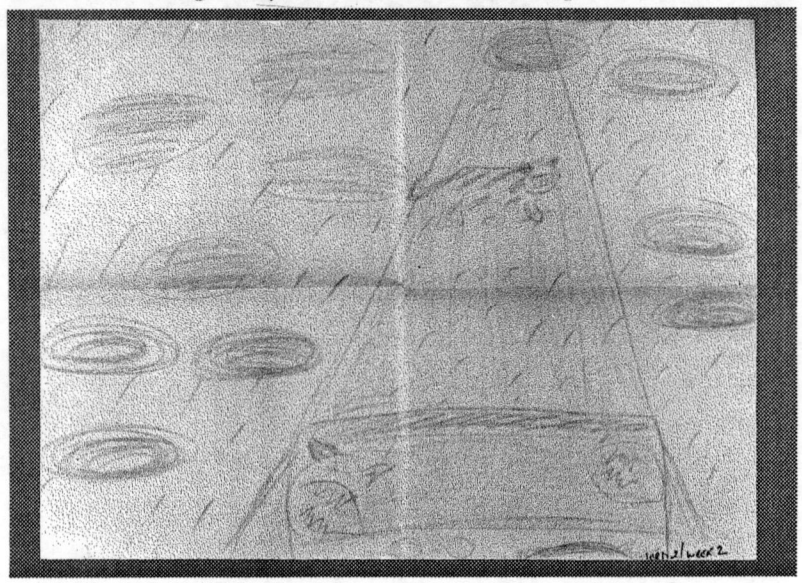

Fig. 16 (p. 141): **Jo: My tigers protect and attack me.**

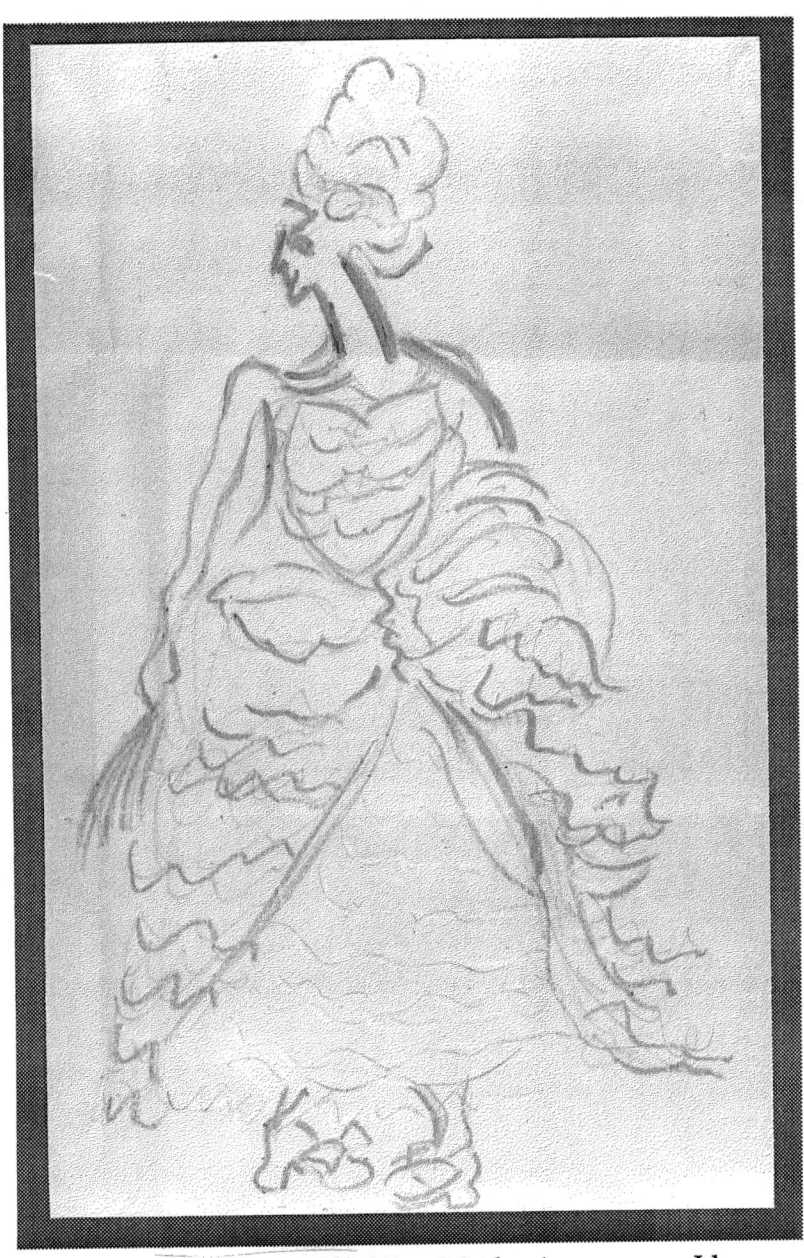

Fig. 18 (pps. 152 & 155): Kim: Mother's message: I love you/I can't love you.

ix

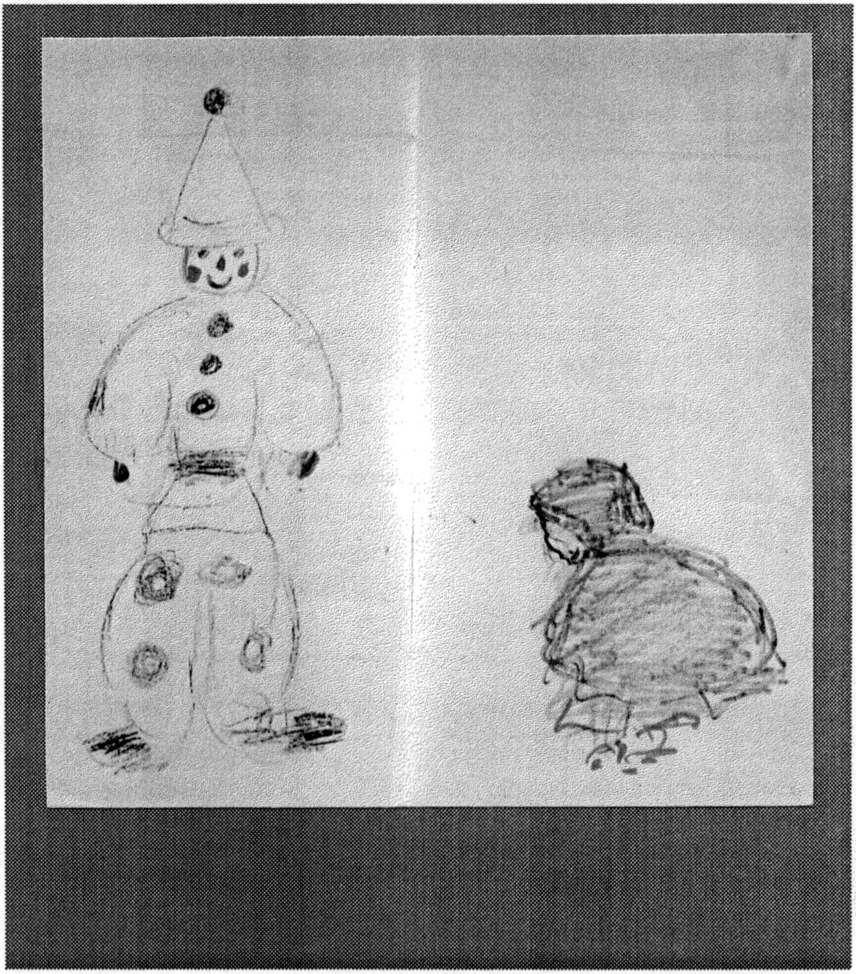

Fig. 19 (p. 153): **Wendy: Red Riding Hood and the clown.**

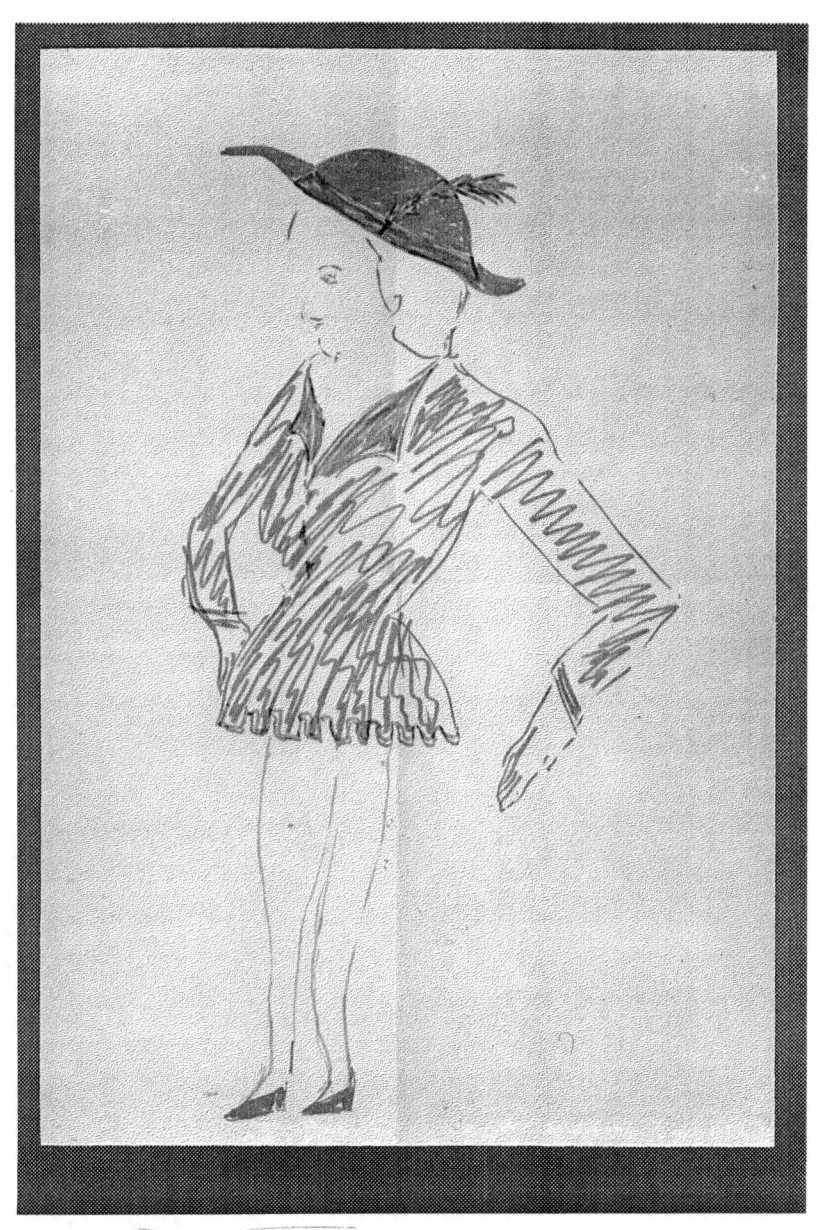

Fig. 20 (pps. 154 & 155): Rosemary: I want to be noticed.

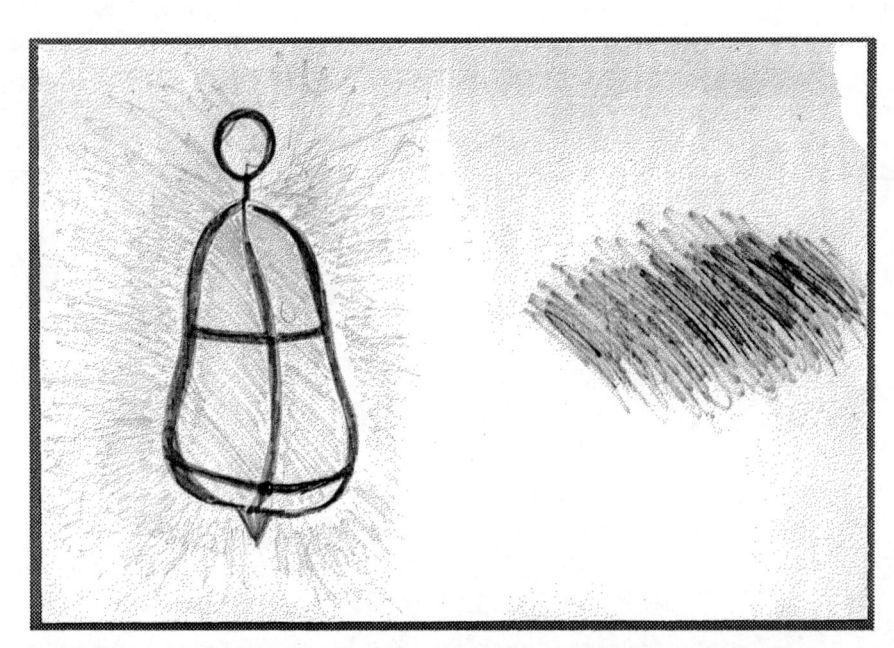

Fig. 21 (pps. 158 & 160): Marianne: Give up fear and see the light

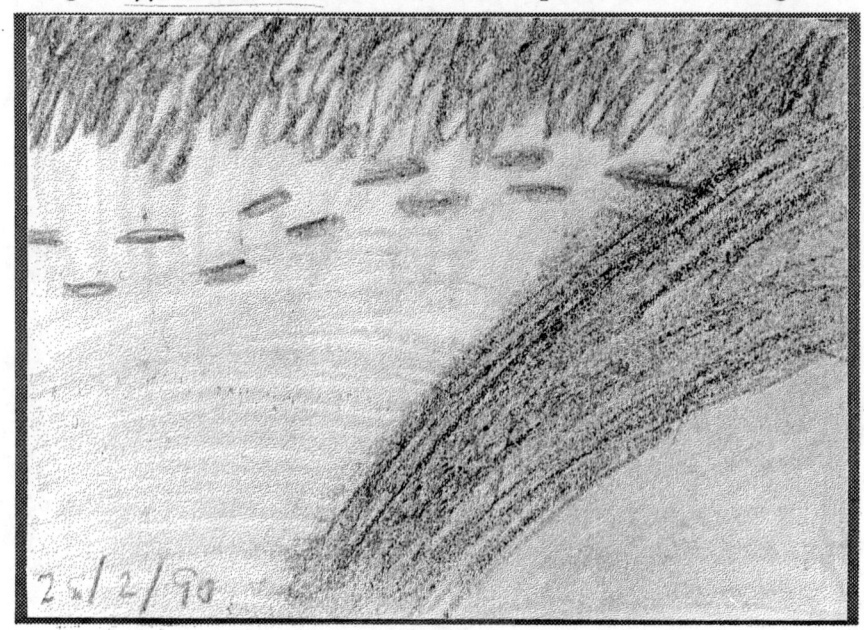

Fig. 22 (p. 169) Jo: The only way is through the sewage.

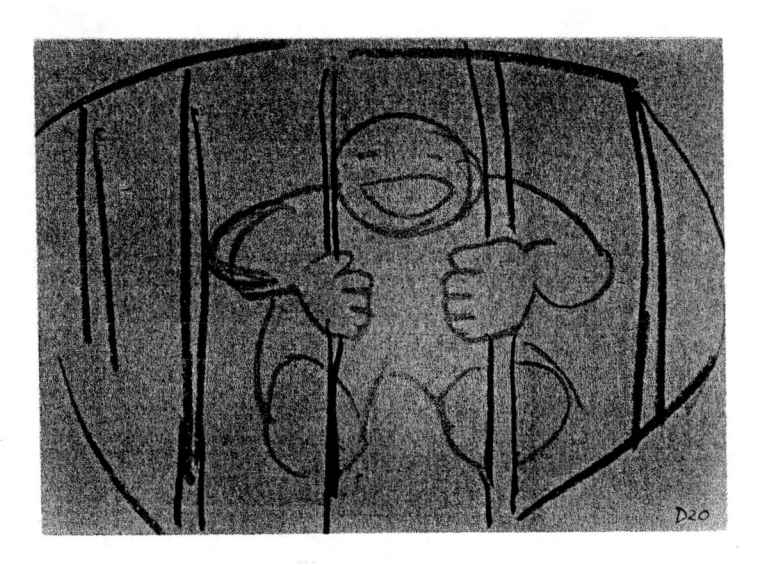

Fig. 23 (p. 170): Kim: I put myself in prison.

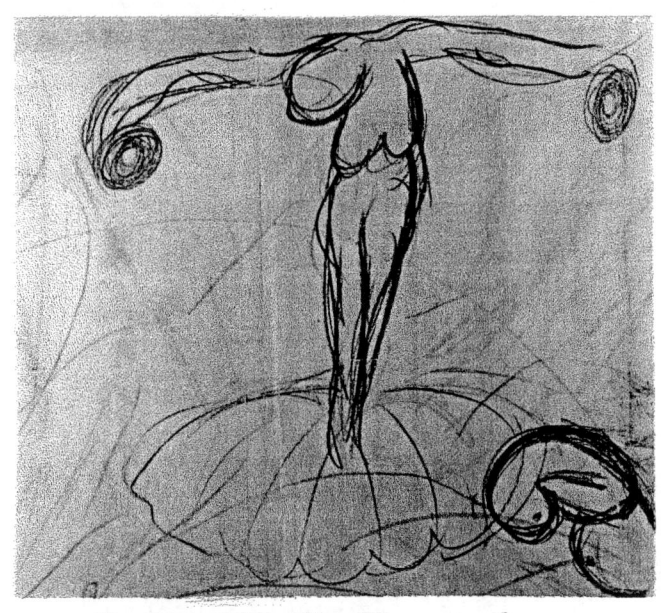

Fig. 26 (p. 180): Kim: Venus on the cross.

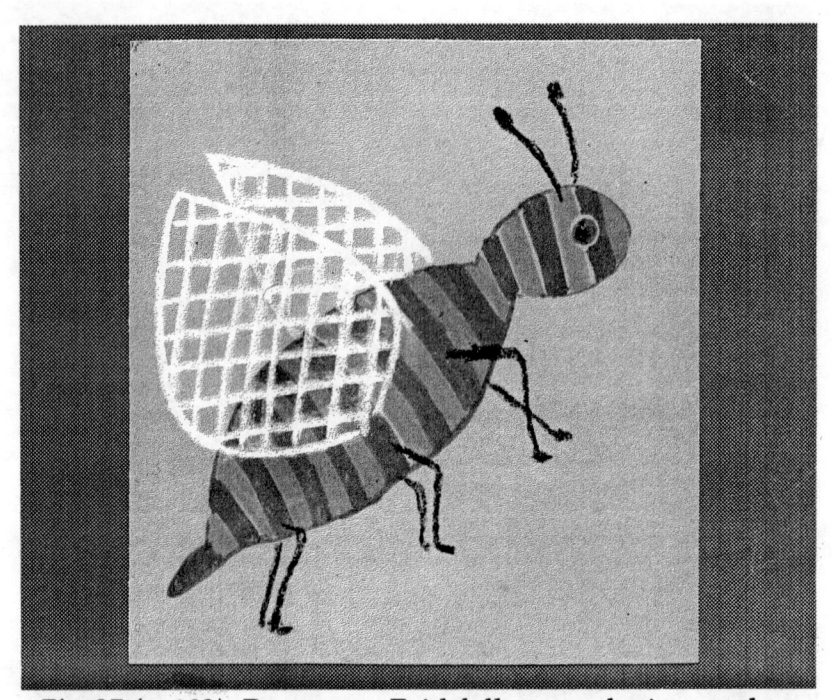

Fig. 27 (p. 183): Rosemary: Faithfully reproducing mother.

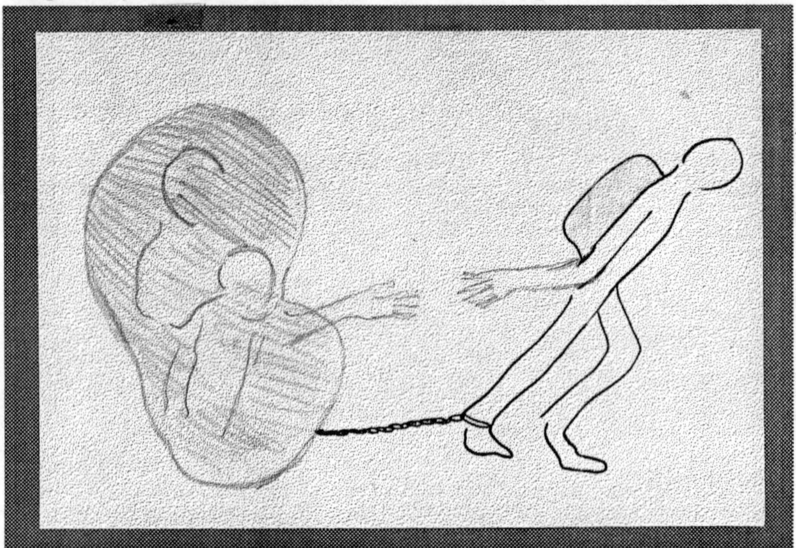

Fig. 28 (p. 184): Marianne: Chain of guilt.

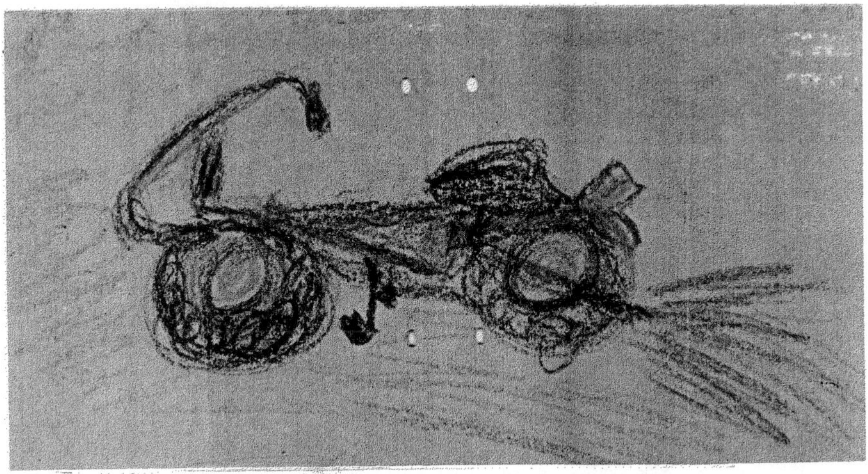

Fig. 29 (p. 193): Brenda: The fantastic bit.

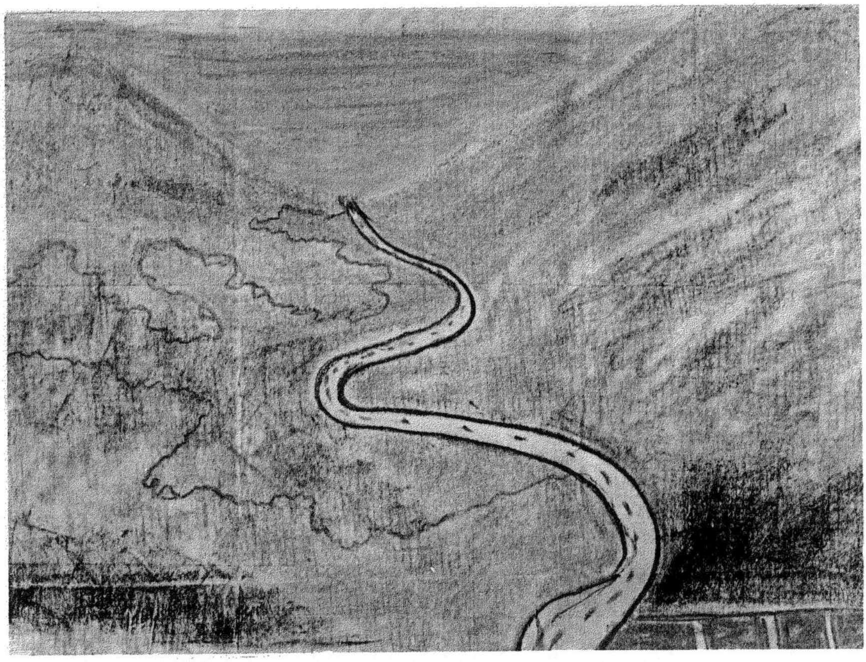

Fig. 30 (p. 194): Rosemary: I'm off the page.

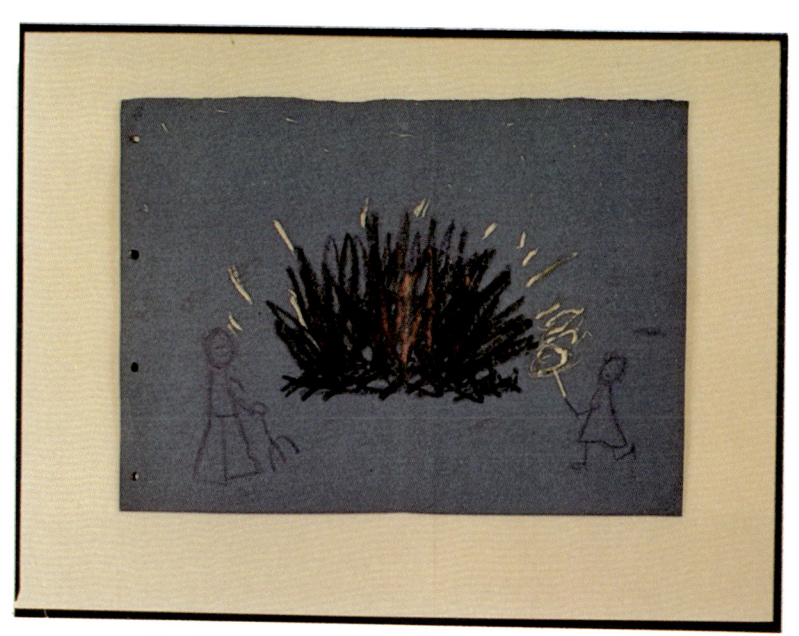

Fig. 10 (pps. 46 & 49): Heather: 'Bonfire Night'.

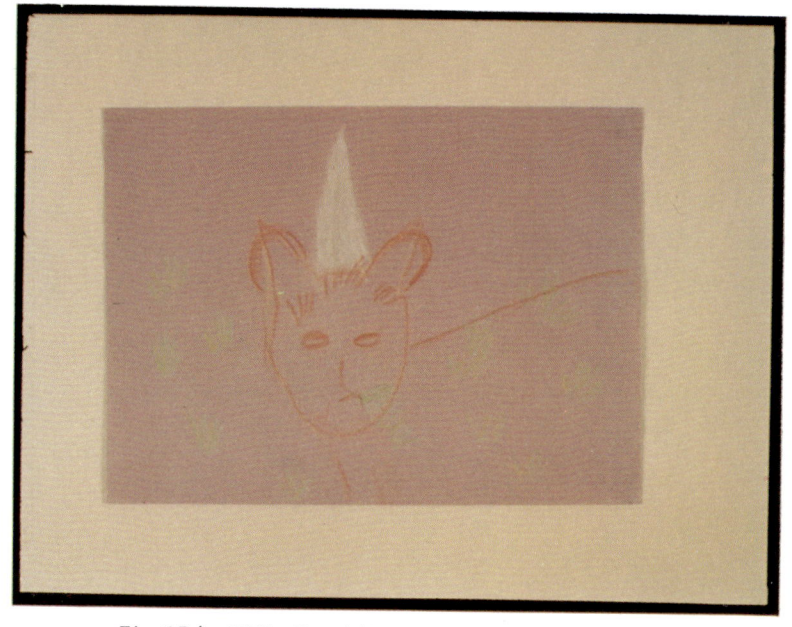

Fig. 15 (p. 139): Geraldine: Goat with unicorn horn.

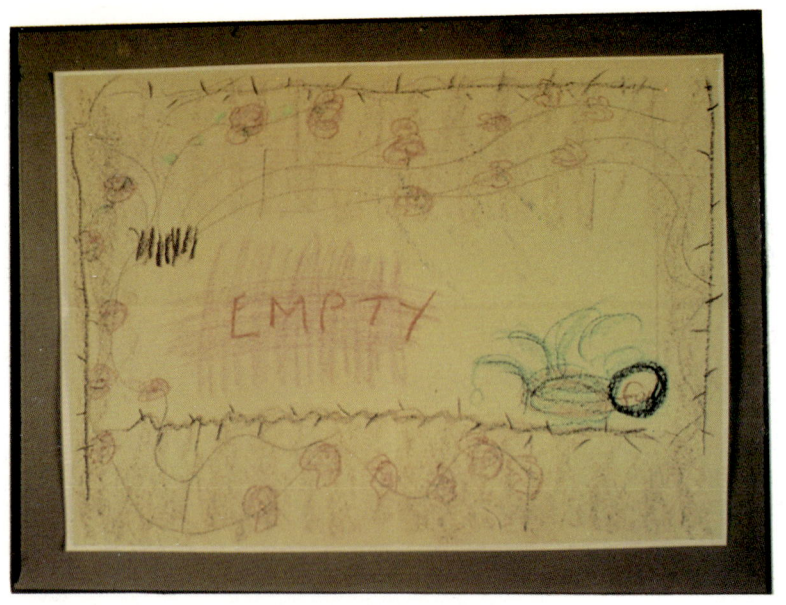

Fig. 17 (p. 146): Jo: Rosebush.

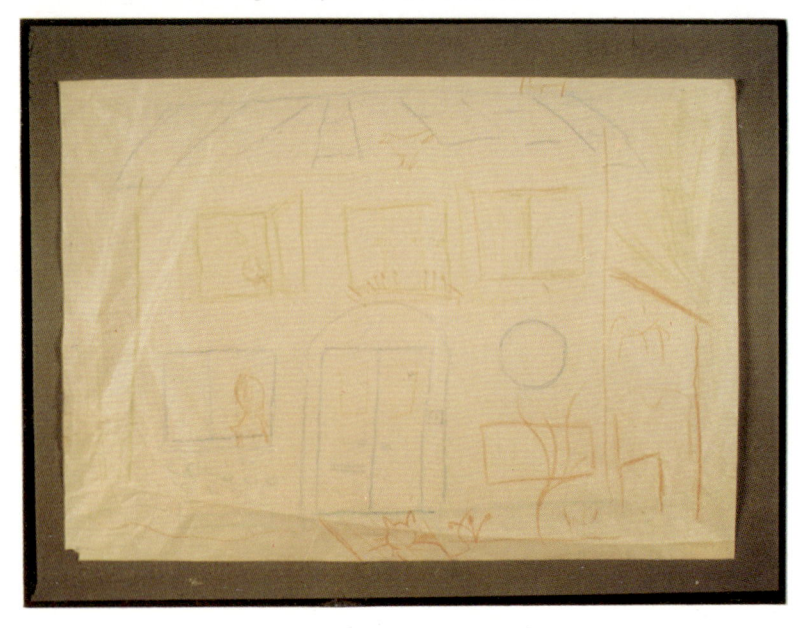

Fig. 31 (pps. 198 & 199): Four people draw a house.

Fig. 24 (p. 175): Nina: Transformation.

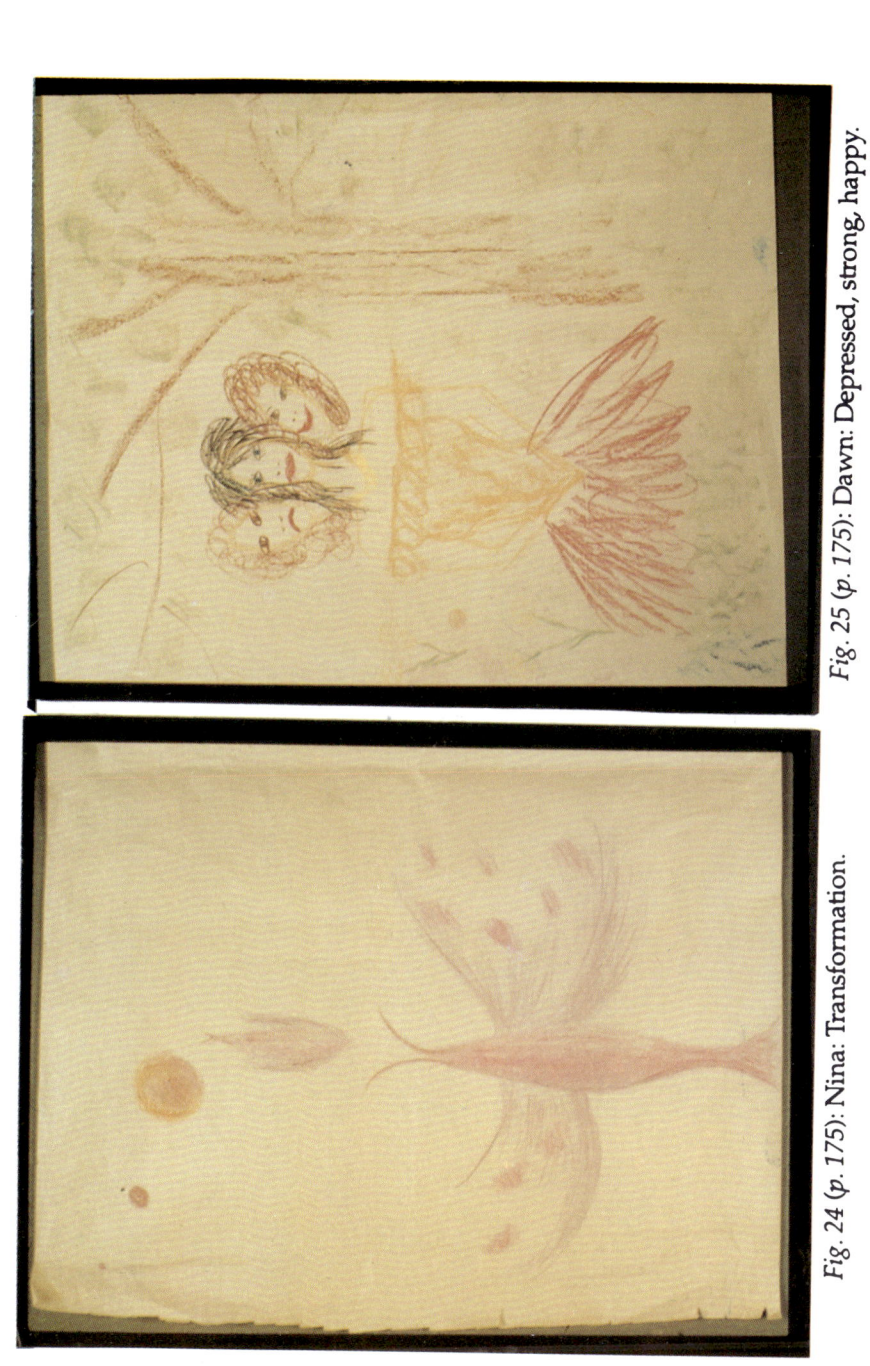

Fig. 25 (p. 175): Dawn: Depressed, strong, happy.

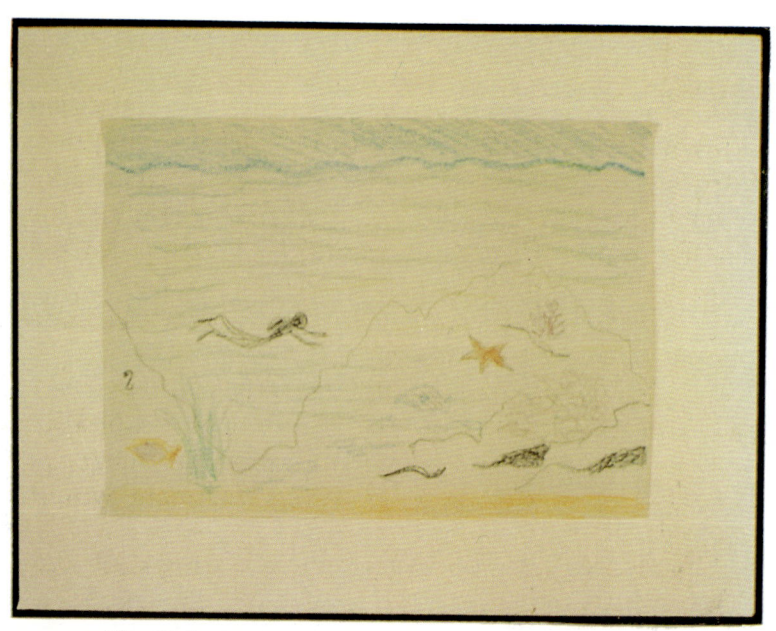

Fig. 32 (p. 211): Marianne: Diving to the unknown.

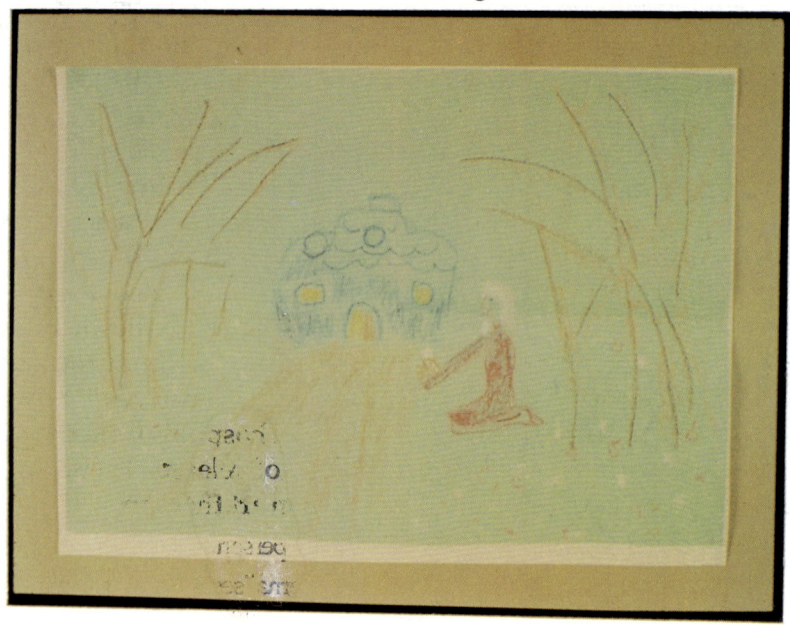

Fig. 33 (p. 215): Rosemary: Teacher of inner wisdom.

xx

I begin:
Last week I shared a poem about taking risks. This applies to the spontaneous, creative process, risking the abandoning of safe familiar thoughts, facing the unknown, where anything may emerge. The gift of risking is the possibility of gaining a valuable insight, valuable for the here and now.

Last week we focused on the creative process. Today we move the focus to art therapy.

Art therapy developed quite recently, mainly since World War II, and was used originally in mental hospitals. Here, often the professional would interpret the image, patient nowhere to be seen; diagnosis and treatment would take into account these interpretations.

Our training in person-centred facilitating skills is a shift away from such practice, enabling the 'patient', the client, to know what the image is about for her, whatever her level of development, of comprehension.

The process of putting down an image spontaneously, in art form, releases, expresses, contains. A child fearful of storms can paint a picture of her fears, discharging her feelings safely, the picture a manageable container. This process in itself can be healing. In the foreword to 'Art as healing', Anthony Stevens says: "By liberating patients from the restrictive confinement of words, and setting loose a much wider vocabulary of paint and clay, Adamson enabled them (the patients) to formulate the meaning to their predicament; and by mobilising the creative resources latent within their own personalities he assisted them to heal themselves." Edward Adamson, an artist working in mental hospitals from the mid-forties, simply allowed this process of release. There can be more: I believe there are four stages in art therapy:

(1) The image manifests itself within the person.
(2) The person conveys that image, externalises it on paper with art material, with clay, however appropriate.

(3) The opportunity, with a facilitator, to dialogue with the picture, so that its meaning might become known on the conscious level.

(4) Then it may be necessary to work on the revealed meaning.

It is my belief that the form of facilitating is imperative: any method which includes judging and interpreting will take the focus away from the client; the meaning of the image will be more about what the counsellor sees than what the client sees. The person-centred approach, based on the belief that the client is trustworthy, response-able, can know best, is more likely to enable the client to know the meaning of the picture for herself. The client can become more autonomous, less dependent in this way, enhancing her self-esteem.

The person-centred approach has the largest amount of evidence— recorded sessions, research etc—of any therapeutic model, showing that personal growth can take place. I am adding to such evidence.

A spontaneous image can contain suppressed material, can have elements of hopes or fears, diverse aspects of the self expressed symbolically, come to us from the subconscious, to be know, to be integrated. It has very much the mysterious, magical quality of dreams—something we fetch up from within, put out there, hardly knowing at first, what it's about. That is why I believe we need to bring a kind of reverence, an awe, to our work with images. They have a kind of aura of the as-yet unknown, requiring our respect.

Art is visible, keepable (unlike words, which we can forget) and can continue to offer up its meaning, when we are ready to know it. We project something significant of ourselves onto the image. And in moments of spontaneous 'Aha!', we know. The person-centred approach, working at the pace of the client, respects that time of readiness—or unreadiness. If the client does not see what the picture shows, at this moment, the counsellor does not push, intrude, rather accepts, lets be, moves on. Perhaps later the client will be ready, will know. Perhaps not.

Working with an image can be safer than talking about me—I am talking about me via the image, a gentler process than 'eyeball to eyeball'. Words become less censored, more spontaneous, 'right side of the brain' words, more likely to contain/reveal pertinent truths. It is safe, as I am likely to see what I am ready to see, at my pace. It is quick; we saw that even in five minutes the essence of meaning can be revealed. Even if it might take rather longer to work on the meaning thus disclosed. Wendy's images tell her she wants more time for herself. She needs to implement that wish now.

Images are a means of communicating for those with limited, or impaired verbal skills, and for the articulate, whose words can distract, defend, deceive. The image is 'spot on'. It can be trusted.

More of this, as we experience for ourselves, in the weeks ahead, with a diversity of art therapy exercises.

Now, to focus on the facilitator: You need to be clear about your purpose; what are you offering, when and why. You have a responsibility to bring material appropriately. You do not begin an exercise fifteen minutes before the end of a session, with inadequate time to deal with the process. Timing is important: when to offer material; is the client— are you!— sufficiently trusting to be open to a new initiative.

If working in a group, allow equal time for sharing to the group members. Be clear and level about your intentions. Don't 'hoodwink' someone into art therapy.

Ensure there will be as little noise as possible, as few interruptions as possible. State to a group that there is to be no talking during the process—talking can shatter the image.

Watch your pace; enough time to close the eyes, relax, quieten, before telling the exercise.

Enough time for the imaging to occur. If offering a guided fantasy, allow sufficient time for each stage. Haste can be very disturbing. Enough time to produce the image.

Now, to the actual person-centred facilitating:

As last term, you are holding up a mirror. Not only to words, but also to the image. You do not lead, direct, interpret. You reflect back the image—the whole process of the image-making, not only the end product.

'You took a piece of paper and folded it in half.'
'You started, turned the paper over, started again.'
'You tore a piece off.'
'You sat with your eyes closed for some minutes before painting.'
'You finished drawing after a few minutes.'

All may be significant for the client. You may reflect size/colour of paper. Kind of material used:

'You used chalk for your mother, felt-tip for you.'

Colour:

'You use the same colour for this whole picture.'
'This is the only part you did in red.'
'You use green for the men in the picture.'
'You put yourself in a different colour to the other people in the picture.'

Position, size:

'You put yourself on the edge of the page.'
'Can you say anything about the size of this shape?'

That which is missing, left out, is often significant:

'There doesn't seem to be a mouth.'
'I notice there are no hands.'
'You have left this part blank.'

Simply point to different aspects, leaving the client as much freedom to respond for herself.

Wider reflections can be fruitful:

'In the last two pictures the eyes are closed, in this picture the eyes are open.'

'You use red for your father each time.'

'You use yellow for the sun and for you.'

'Tentative phrases are helpful—"it seems as if", "perhaps", "maybe", "it looks as if"—implying you're not dogmatic, allowing the client to firm up for herself.'

With images, identifying is even more likely than with words: images can be very emotive. A certain image may ring bells for *you*. Be careful not to tip your material onto the client. Notice what's yours, put it aside, be there for the client. It is not *your* picture.

It is useful looking at a series of images, to see if similar themes are emerging, or what.

As the picture is a projection, an extension of some aspect of the self made visible, it is valid to try and make 'bridges' between the picture and the person, so the link might be known. However well you work with the picture, if you treat it as something separate from the person, you are not working to full effect. So:

'This stag is in Scotland. 'Does that ring bells for you, Scotland?'

'My grandfather was Scottish.'

'Is that significant for you at present?'

'I've been on a visit to my family in South Africa. I need to know I have roots here too.'

'I need to define the shape of *this* cat.'

'Can you associate with that?' Defining the shape of the cat?'

'Oh yes! I need to define the shape of this cat. Me!'

As you become more sure, you will work ever more spontaneously, creatively, working with *all* the material before you, as it presents itself. The client—maybe you need to reflect voice, body posture, expression, words—the picture, and the link between the two. Give full attention to feelings at any time.

So, it is a creative process for both the client and the counsellor, as you both set forth on a journey into the unknown, trusting your sense of intuitive knowing, where the focus is at any moment on that unfolding process. The more you give yourself up to the moment, the more you suspend your own need to know and judge and think, the more likely you are to enable the client to grasp the meaning of her image to the full.

There are those who believe that only verbal reflecting counts as person-centred counselling, that including art deviates, reduces, is something other. I disagree: The image being a projection of the self in symbolic form, to include it as part of the person, to dialogue with it in a person-centred way, seems most valid.

Evidence tells me that verbal and non-verbal intelligence is required for integration and growth, and art therapy, leading to the right side of the brain knowing leads to such integration, wholeness.

I came to see that in talking about the image, the client speaks more spontaneously, words transform to 'right side of the brain' words, of equal existential in-the-now import as the image, containing uncensored truths. When these are reflected along with the images, much awareness can occur. In fact, it is my belief that far more needs to be done in counselling training to incorporate this spontaneous wisdom with the use of the creative therapies. Integrated counsellor training leading to integrated clients.

An exciting business!

Now it's time for you to have another taster. We'll do an art therapy exercise: I suggest I demonstrate with someone, say, for about five minutes, then anyone can come in with facilitating comments for five minutes, and then we'll have learning and process comments. The remaining time you could go into threes—clients, counsellor, observer—to work on your images. The observer will write down feedback for the counsellor during the session, then give it to the counsellor who will write it down, as useful feedback. I suggest ten minutes for each corner—five minutes counselling, five minutes feedback—and that leaves us ten minutes when we can come together for any sharing. And we finish with the usual ten minutes monitoring of the session.

The students agree to this suggestion.

Exercise with image 12—an animal
'Make yourself comfortable—
close your eyes—
relax—
breathe easy, regular breaths— 'push aside your thoughts—quieten—
—now—
—without censoring—
let an image come up for you—of an animal ———
(pause about 2 minutes)
—when you're ready, open your eyes gently — and convey your
image on paper, however you want—
when they all have paper and colours
—you have about 5-7 minutes—'
Later: 'you have a minute or two to finish'.

When they stop, I ask: 'Who wants to share their picture with me?' It's Geraldine. I say that I realise, when I demonstrate for such a short time, I tend to go more quickly than 'usual', to show as much as I can. Someone keeps time for us for 5 minutes.

We sit side by side—the picture in front of us.

G: What came up quite spontaneously was a goat.

L: A goat (*I reflect back*).

G: Yes, eating grass. What came up most prominently was his horn.

L: The horn is most prominent; it's a 'he' goat eating grass. (*I reflect back*).

G: I'm surprised—yes.

L: You're surprised?

L: And the most prominent feature is his horn. Any idea what that might be about?

G: It might be about—something magical, like a unicorn.

L: So the goat has some sort of magical aspect—can you link with that in any way? (*I make a 'bridge' to Geraldine*).

G: Perhaps mystery.

L: Mystery?

G: Mmm…(*pause*).

L: Can you say any more about mystery?

G: Shakes her head.

L: What about the way you've done the mouth? (*I work on the picture*).

G: It's chewing the grass. I didn't want to draw the body.

L: So you've just indicated the body here, mainly it's the head.

G: Yes…

L: It's a goat, with a sketchy body, chewing grass, and with a magical horn. (*I sum up*)—can you make any links at all? (*Bridge*).

G: When the goat came up, I didn't want a goat, it's silly, but it kept being there.

L: So you don't think much of a goat.

G: —it's silly.

L: It's silly.

G: Yes…

L: Silly and magical. (*Wider reflection*). Does that ring bells for you? (*bridge*)

G: Hmm…

L: I notice there are no pupils in the eyes (*a missing bit*).

G: —no. The focus is on this aimless chewing.

L: So; sketchy body, no pupils, a silly goat, aimless chewing, and a unicorn—Hmm…(*pause*) (*wait, at the pace of client*) —and you've done the ears pointed, and then round—(*to the picture*)

G: The round ears are too much like a cat, so I changed them to look more like a goat.

L: You wanted the goat to have goat's ears—not cat's, does that say anything for you? Changing the ears?

G: I'm always changing something in me.

L: And ears?

G: Changing the way I'm hearing...

L: Hearing?

G: Listening to me perhaps, yes...

L: Listening to yourself...

L: And you give the goat goat's ears, and yet here's this horn which is not like a goat's.

G: Like a unicorn—with magical qualities.

L: So the goat also has magical qualities of a unicorn—does that speak to you?

G: It's far less mysterious now that I've talked about it.

L: It is?

G: —

L: And this?

G: Grass all around, for my aimless eating.

L: Your aimless eating.

G: Yes...

L: So you're eating aimlessly, and you've hardly put in the body. (*Wider reflection*).

G: I was worried about the body, not showing it up.

L: Are you worried about *your* body, not showing it up?

G: I hide my body. I worry, I eat, and then I want to hide my body. So I hide it under loose clothing. *See Fig. 15. (Colour)*

On several occasions I reflected back, and Geraldine chose not to take the reflection further. My job, simply, to hold the mirror up; to respect what the client sees, or what, at present, she does not wish to see. I could say: 'I notice you don't respond to...' That, too, is holding up the mirror.

The other students come in, but I can't hear it on the tape-recorder: very frustrating.

139

Geraldine says she's got a lot, about her over-eating, conforming. She's excited about the unicorn aspect, even if she doesn't quite understand it yet. Or what 'he' means.

I say some aspects may have got overlooked, go unexplored. Yet, in five minutes, much has come up.

The students go into 'three's; to share the remaining pictures, practice, receive feedback. I ask if I can join as observer.

Geraldine is counsellor for Dawn.

Dawn talks of her frustration at work.

Geraldine: 'Are you getting your needs met?' (*Away from 'frustration*).

Jo—as observer—gives feedback here: this was directive, out of context. Dawn says the intervention jarred. I ask Geraldine what was she investing in that intervention for herself?

Marianne draws a black cat: 'Live, warm, affectionate, blissed out.' She wants to be more like the cat. A hope. Kim reflects back words well, doesn't make links with image.

The students monitor. We end.

Later, Rosemary writes: 'I produce an image of a soft white fluffy cat, stretched out in bright sunshine. During the reflection I realise that I find it difficult to relax, that I need to do it more. When I relax I feel I ought to be doing something—this is an internalised voice of my mother telling me that it is wrong to do nothing. From the reflections provided of my cat image, I see that being too busy fits my mother better than me. When I'm too busy I become ill. I must listen to my body—and my cat.'

Here, the image, a hope, a wish, needing attention.

Heather: ' A stag with beautiful branched antlers, standing proudly, in the hills of Scotland. I remember previous images: crown of thorns, paper hat, now antlers, all above my head. What does it mean? Crown of thorns—antlers stretching up—the spiritual aspect; paper hat, part of my past which was put on me; the antlers—strong, positive, me growing up. I felt disappointed that I couldn't reproduce the beautiful stag on paper. A wider reflection was made about inside/outside: often I'm sure inside (the beautiful strong stag), but how to convey this out there?'

Jo writes: 'I drew a road with a pit, me in a car, and an angry tiger between the pit and the car. Geraldine asked about the snarling tiger. I realised the animals are attacking me—just as last week I was caning me. My internal censors, when I am full of fear what to do. As Geraldine probed, I felt anger about how I've voluntarily made myself poor in order not to be a wage slave. Feelings of total lack of confidence overwhelmed me—very new for me to let such feelings through—and the loss brought about by Sophie's death—feeling totally alone. So; pitfalls everywhere, one on my road—one tiger-part of me to protect me, the other tiger-part can attack me when I least expect it.' See Fig. 16.

Comments

In this session I gave some theory about art therapy, and some guidelines for person-centred facilitating, to focus on the terms ahead. 'Talking about' only becomes relevant when, in subsequent weeks, students make the discoveries for *themselves* when *they* facilitate, when *they* are given feedback. When, from the 'client's' seat, *they* discover what kind of intervention is helpful or unhelpful. When, as 'observer' *they* can see what works, what moves on, what jars!

To me, 'talking about' on its own is inadequate for real learning.

I 'demonstrated' with Geraldine—to enact some of these guidelines. Then it is over to the students. Three relevant stages in experiential learning: theory, demonstration, experience. Geraldine again learned about the spontaneous, creative process: at first she didn't know what the image meant. Then, having aspects of the picture reflected to her—simply reflected to her; no judgment, no interpretation—she was able to make some connections for herself. So, evidence of the validity of the person-centred way.

I must watch my pace when I demonstrate—no need to impress/amaze, show all. Slow down to my usual counselling speed. I'll show more!

This session was a microcosm of person-centred teaching; first theory, then an opportunity for students to discover the theory for themselves, then, to apply it elsewhere.

It seems to me that with images, students are able to connect, re-discover their right side of the brain intelligence. That's what it's all about.

Reference: Edward Adamson: Art as healing.

Application

In any training session and course where imaging, the creative spontaneous process, intuition, and art is valued as a means towards growth in personal development.

Where complementing and balancing the area of words, thoughts, and intellect with non-verbal knowing is seen as important in the integration of the person and in the learning process. Be it a child with emotional difficulties, a trainee at an occupational training centre, an AIDS sufferer, a drug addict, a victim of rape, a depressed patient, a survivor of every kind of trauma, a couple, a family needing to relate better, a management team wanting to explore its dynamic, a person in therapy with repressed fear, grief or pain, a person needing to re-connect with love, affirmation and spirituality—person-centred art therapy can lead to release, healing and growth.

SESSION FIFTEEN
More experiential learning:
Exercise with image—a rose bush

"I expressed more of myself in one day of painting than I had in a year of talking about myself in words."

Janie Rhyne

Purpose

For students to experience tapping into the spontaneous world of images, and to become aware of material contained therein which needs to be known. The subconscious speaking to us of issues we avoid, deny to our consciousness, but which are necessary for integration.

For students to practice person-centred skills—'holding up the mirror' to the picture, allowing the client to see the meaning.

To notice how they sabotage themselves as facilitators; what gets in the way.

For students to give one another level feedback, to learn from one another.

To discover for themselves the immediacy, and accuracy of images. That, with images, we reach awareness more quickly than with words. That images keep, the process of discovery can continue.

To begin to see how creative is the facilitating process—being in the moment, now with the image, now the words, the tone, the body-language, now linking with an earlier session, or picture — floating spontaneously, wherever the focus is in the moment. So, both client and counsellor, tapping ever more into 'right side of the brain'—the world, not of thinking, but of knowing.

Nina is away (having her baby).
Marianne is at home with an ill child.
We are eight.

Exercise with image 13—a rose bush
I offer another art therapy exercise. I say something like:
  Close your eyes—relax—push aside your thoughts — And now—see what image emerges for you—of a rose bush—what kind of a bush—notice the details — where is it—look about you — what time of year — day — what's the weather like — Be aware of everything about this rose bush — (4 or so minutes).
  —and now, in your own time, open your eyes, and put your image on paper. (7 or so minutes).

Jo wants to talk about her picture. We decide to work with her as a group.

L: I noticed you started with brown, all the way around (*reflect process of picture making*).

J: Yes, it's a walled garden.

L: So you put the wall in first.

J: I put the wall in first.

W: What's that on the wall? (*reflects picture*)

J: That's barbed wire. I put barbed wire on top of it. No way out.

M: No way out. Barbed wire on the wall.

(*No comment to this...*)

J: The rose bush is here, moving away from the base, moving along the wall, taking the wall over.

L: So here's the wall and the rose grows along, takes it over. How does this speak to you, Jo: there's no way out, and the rose takes over the wall. (*Wider reflection and 'bridge'*).

J: That's the contradiction I live with: on the one side things look very black, and on the other side I know it's starting to change. The image came quite spontaneously. Over here, this is water, gushing out of the ground, almost volcanic water.

D: After you completed drawing the wall you did the water, before you did the rose. (*Sequence of the picture making*).

K: The water is coming out, gushing out. (*No time for Jo to respond to above*).

J: Uncontrollable, volcanic.

L: Is there something uncontrollable coming out of you? (*Making a 'bridge'*)

J: Yes—it's not lava, it's water.

L: Water.

J: Yes.

R: So after the volcanic water you did the rose, at the opposite end of the water, and moving away from the base, towards the water, along the wall.

J: And also, this is a cropped rose bush which has been cut off and is starting to grow again.

L: Have you been cut off and are starting to grow again? (*Bridge*)

J: Yes.

L: I'm a cut off rose bush starting to grow again away from my base towards some gushing water.

G: What are these? (*Again, no time for J to respond to the above summary*)

J: The roses. I kept on thinking how tiny and frail they were and that nothing could stop them.

K: And this—(*points*).

(*Bridge re roses might have been helpful: stay with pace of client*)

J: This is an empty space in the middle. This is exactly how I feel—I write 'empty' and then I try and cover up that I've written it. I have an ambivalence—I'm ashamed to admit that I'm empty.

G: You're talking about determination (*avoids shame about being empty—rescues again*).

J: It's more that something is happening that I have no control over.

(*This emotive phrase could have been reflected*)

R: And the roses are unstoppable.

J: Yes.

R: You've done the roses the same colour as you used for covering up 'empty'. (*Wider reflection of colour*)

J: Yes. (*Doesn't expound*)

L: And the leaves:

J: A few little leaves, poor things.
L: What's that about?
J: My flamboyance. I could be more flamboyant.
R: You've done the stems the same colour as the barbed wire.
(*Wider reflection of colour*)
J: Yes. (*Jo hasn't taken this up. Still a good reflection. Perhaps a 'bridge' here*)
R: What time of year is it?
J: Early summer, after the winter.
D: Do you feel 'after the winter'?
J: I'm in winter—I find this quite a hopeful drawing.
R: I see you've chosen green paper.
J: Yes, that's fertile.
L: What's fertile for you?
J: I'm feeling very black—so this is hopeful.
L: So it's something about the hope of early 'summer' to come.
K: You've written 'full' in the water, and 'empty' here.
J: It's the empty that upsets me. It's wrong to be empty. I try to obliterate it. I'm ashamed.
L: Is that what you do with shame—cover it up?
J: Yes.
R: I notice the water is a long way from the rose—the rose is getting close to the water.
J: Yes, I feel very hopeful. The rose is tenacious.
L: The water and the cut down bit of the rose: you went over it several times.
J: That is the split in me: the cut down bit and the gushing water, but also, I'd have to be killed in order to stop me flowing.
R: I notice the cut down bush is the same colour as the barbed wire.
J: It's the same thing really. I am the wall. And I am the rose inside the wall. *See Fig. 17. (Colour)*

We comment:
Kim is aware she came in too quickly—before Jo had been able to respond to a reflection. Pace is important: to be at the pace of the client, to let her respond before moving on.

Good use of 'wider reflections': same colour of stem—colour of barbed wire—colour of buds, and obliterating 'empty'—one or two directive comments:

'Water far away from the rose'—let the client describe, get there first.'.

Geraldine reflected: 'Determination'. Jo says no—she hadn't used that word. What was Geraldine's agenda to introduce the word at that point?

The importance of 'bridges'—linking key issues to the person; after all, the picture is an extension of the person—if you work with it as something separate, the client may not hear its message.

The students decide to work, as a group, with the remaining images. I observe.

To summarise:

Geraldine has a diagonal line; on one side a 'barren, neglected, isolated' bush, on the other a bush in full bloom with many roses, warm and nurtured.

Heather draws a rose from childhood—mother told her its name is 'peace'. Mother, and rose, in same colours.

Dawn draws a bush with one central rose—weeds are overtaking it. She cries: it's about work—she must leave, can't take any more, is forever strong, giving, finds it hard to be vulnerable, ask for help. Now she allows herself to cry.

Rosemary writes: 'I produce a rose bush with seven colours on it, in early summer, some roses in full bloom, others in bud, a waterfall reaching the roots. Seven colours? Probably to do with not excluding any colours—opportunities. (Here I thought of the seven colours of the rainbow—that's *my* thought, not Rosemary's, saying something to *me*.) The waterfall? To nourish my roots, for my growth. The season? This summer, the first for many years not spoiled by exams. The roses—some in full bloom, some buds? Aspects of myself, my potential.'

Jo adds: I am gradually beginning to understand the importance in counselling of not asking leading questions.

I no longer feel I have to explain what is in the drawing, for in fact I don't know myself until the counselling is under way. A very useful session and I felt astonished that my unconscious self, when allowed to speak, does allow through a lot of hopeful growth which is totally cut off from my conscious mind.

Comments

How quickly the central issue emerges! Let your intuitive ears pick it up.

For Jo, the ambivalence of being walled in, and growing. Now she needs to work on the issue. Working with the image may not be the whole of the work, but a vital part of it, revealing that which is needed to be done for integration.

Some students are away: when you miss a session of an experiental course, you can ask someone what took place, but you can't regain the experience—it's gone. No notes to copy. You've missed YOUR perception. Perhaps this effects, in part, the high level of attendance.

Application

Again, can be used in training and education, and in counselling, therapy, group therapy, art therapy, with terminally ill, with addicts, for self help groups—all settings where human development is important.

In the ensuing weeks there follow a variety of art therapy exercises. Each offers the potential for whatever is being suppressed at that moment, to surface, be seen and be recognised—important information needed on the road to integration. Each exercise can be adapted and offered in a wide range of situations in order to bring unaware aspects to awareness.

SESSION SIXTEEN
Guided fantasy: costume room

"A broader view of art therapy is our plea, to stop being bound only by the concepts and interpretations of psychoanalytic theory, and to move into a higher self-actualising level of approach, i.e. into the potential of creativity as the agent of change in restoring and maintaining mental health."

Mary Lee Hodnett

Purpose

To learn about guided fantasy.
To experience for oneself, with a guided fantasy, what image can emerge.
To practice person-centred facilitating, to see what the image can reveal.
To give and receive feedback.

Nina had a baby girl—is away today.

I say about recording a session for the portfolio: As 'client', it is not enough to say what the picture revealed to you. You need to indicate what the 'counsellor' did (what did she reflect, was she non-directive, in tune with you, or what?) and how you responded/felt as a result.

Exercise with image 14—Guided fantasy: a costume room
We decide on this format:
One person shares her image in the group for 7 minutes—half the group counselling, half observing. We have feedback. Then we repeat this process with another person, counsellors and observers switching role. We break into triads to work with the remaining pictures and come back together for feedback in the whole group. I say what I mean by a guided fantasy.

I tell a story (the 'guided, bit). You fantasise around it, go with it, or not, whatever is spontaneous and appropriate for you. The purpose of a guided fantasy—(as of every art therapy exercise)—is to stop you thinking, judging; to move you from left side of brain, to right, where you can allow a story in images, symbolic parts of you to emerge.

Now:

Close your eyes ——— and now—you're in the costume room of a theatre—looking about you—at the rows of costumes, the hats, shoes, whatever you see— As you look about you, you may be drawn to one costume in particular — have a good look at it — note all the details — what are you doing—feeling—and when you're ready, open your eyes—and make visible, however you need to do it, your time in the costume room.

As they begin to draw: 'You have some 7 minutes.' Later: 'You've 2-3 minutes left.

Kim talks about her picture:

K: It's a gold, frilly costume.

J: Does that speak to you?

K: No.

(*Jo made a 'bridge'—that's OK, whether at that moment Kim can make a connection or not.*)

K: She's looking over her shoulder.

J: And the hair?

(*Here Jo could have stayed with the previous statement: 'Looking over her shoulder.' It's important to stay in tune with the client rather than pursue one's own path.*)

K: It's my mother—her look.

Rosemary: Can you say something about how you coloured the dress.

(*Here again, Rosemary could have stayed with: 'It's my mother.' There's more here!*)

Geraldine: Can you say more about your mother (*brings her back*), her look?

K: It's her look: a mixed message: 'Come here, I love you,' and: 'I can't love you, you haven't done what I want.'

Marianne: What about the gold colour?

(*Again, stay with previous comment.*)

It's not enough to reflect accurately, you need to stay with, be intuitively in tune with the client, the client's pace *your* pace. Very soon you can intuit what the main issue is, for Kim today: her feelings about the mother. And to work with the image more: 'Looking over her shoulder,' point to that part of the picture, the neck, the shoulder, which Kim drew more heavily than the rest.

The two statements—'looking over her shoulder' and 'it's my mother, her look'—were the big ones to develop. Wider reflection to Kim's previous pictures about her mother would be helpful. We need to transmogrify our ears from thinking ears to knowing ears; to KNOW what it's about, to focus on that. Right-side of the brain—ears!

This takes much time, much practice, much personal work. I am not criticising; the students are doing well on their path. I am pointing to the way ahead.

Kim's picture showed how quickly the message can emerge. *See Fig. 18.*

The students are reflecting better, though not always in harmony with the client.

Wendy shares her picture:

W: Two images came—the clown on one side, Red-riding-hood on the other. I put them both in.

Kim: You're laughing.

W: It's a cover up.

Heather: A cover up?

W: I'm unable to make up my mind as usual.

Dawn: As usual?

Kim: The clown is much larger than little Red-riding-hood (*an interpretation. No time for W to respond to D*).

W: No. The clown is stronger (*an open-ended comment about the clown and little Red-riding-hood would leave W. free to give the quality for herself.*)

Heather: How have you drawn Red-riding-hood?

W: The hood is important.

152

Heather: The hood.
W: Red.
Dawn: Red?
W: I'm not keen on red.

Good reflecting. Not enough work on the image: clown has smiling face—Red-riding-hood has no features. Her cloak is coloured in—the only coloured-in part of the picture. Associate with: not being able to make up her mind; anything like that now?
Associate: Clown. Red-riding-Hood. Hood. What do they mean for Wendy? *See Fig. 19.*

Sometimes the client is not ready to see what there is to see. That's OK. The person-centred approach is respectful, stays at the client's pace. But if the counsellor isn't able to see what there is to see, that may prevent/delay the client from seeing. Sometimes her own identifying may get in the way, needs acknowledging in supervision.

Rosemary shares her picture in the triad. I've asked if I can join, as observer. Jo is her counsellor.

R: This is a sort of Robin Hood-Maid Marion kind of costume. Principal man in pantomime.

J: Pantomime?

(To select just one word from the sequence can skew it. 'Principal man' was part of that phrase, also: Maid Marion—and pantomime. All of possible significant to R).

Often all is said in the first minute of the session. This might be such a microcosm.

R: I wanted a body—my legs are in there.

J: Your legs are visible.

(Visible has different quality to 'in there'—paraphrase can verge on interpretation. Half the phrase omitted: 'I wanted a body.')

J: You concentrate on this part of the body (—*indicates torso, as against legs.*)

(Very directive, interpretive. R. couldn't respond.)

R: I want to show that I'm there (*more of the same theme*).

J: The underneath coming through.

(*An interpretation; rather than reflecting what's given—I want to show I'm there.*)

J: Can you say more about Maid Marion?

R: I'm not sure.

J: You're ambivalent (*interpretation—not the same as 'I'm not sure*).

J: What about the colour (*working with the picture*).

R: I don't wear red, I wear green.

J: You look good in green (*interpretation*).

J: What about the hat?

R: I started with the hat. It's meant to be jaunty—it's more like a horrible school hat.

(*Association would be helpful here—also: she started with the hat—in red—she doesn't like red—wider reflection.*) See Fig. 20.

Jo reflects well at times, interprets at times. Her pace is too fast. She dashes from one aspect to the next, not hearing the issue emerge: 'I want to show that I'm here, I want attention.' Once you have the feel of the issue, you can focus on it, no need to dash elsewhere.

Geraldine has made some 'mind-blowing' (her phrase) connection—from the goat which turns into a unicorn (two weeks ago), to the fairy with a magic wand today. She says she'll share later. (Does not do so.)

Marianne doesn't know what her image means (a sheepskin coat). Sometimes we don't know. The image keeps—we may know later, see further. Or it could be an image about something yet to come.

Last year, one student didn't want a costume. She wanted to be herself. She could not understand the picture. On the way out she said she'll be away next week, she's going with her husband to a conference to do with his work.

I say: Is there a link with your picture?

She says: *Yes!* I find it hard to be myself in such a situation. The picture is telling me now, preparing me; BE YOURSELF! How helpful! I'll take it with me.'

Some students at times are still counsellor centred; thinking about *their* intervention, rather than in tune with the client, making interventions appropriate to the client at any moment, letting go of their own agenda.

Rosemary writes:
'I was shown by Jo that certain parts of the body were more important than others. However, she used the term 'visible' which was a theme that applied to her own image (identification projection. L.) and I couldn't own it as mine. She failed to pick up on the phrases which were important, such as 'principal man' and 'family'.

It was in the feedback from Liesl to Jo that my image became meaningful to me—I want to be noticed, show 'I am there'. It shows the difference between skilled facilitating and those of us who are still learning.'

Kim writes:
'I chose a golden sparkling costume as I would imagine Marie Antoinette must have worn. My mother is wearing the costume. Her head is turned in a characteristic manner. She is beautiful. The only bit of 'reality' is in the shoes. The shoes are *me!* They are the reality. The ugliness.

Only I know her ugliness, duplicity, mixed messages.' *See Fig. 18.*

Comments

In this session the students:

Could tap into their creative process and fetch up an image. The less you know what it means initially, the more material is likely to emerge. If we know—it could be the thinking mode. Not knowing: trust the intuition, the subconscious—what is it wanting me to know?

They are making strides in empathic listening, in paraphrasing.

They need to work more with the image, stay at the client's pace, make 'bridges' from image to person, make wider links, and be aware of the emerging theme. Early days!

The landscape is not flat: there are mountains, hills, valleys and plains. As with counselling, we reflect certain aspects more than others, feeling words being the mountains in the landscape.

I'm excited: I've opened the door to the image world, and I am able to watch what people make of it. What a privilege!

Application

As before:
  In training.
The exercise can be used one-to-one, or with groups in a variety of therapeutic and educational settings.

SESSION SEVENTEEN
More practice: Magic Gift Shop

"It was not until I started to experiment with spontaneous painting that I was first able to gain access to the undistorted reality of my childhood."

Alice Miller 'The drama of being a child'

Purpose

Each week I offer a different art therapy exercise. One aim is, to give a variety of experiences, which the students can adapt for use in their diverse work settings.

Another aim, perhaps less obvious though more central, is to give opportunity for practice. Both the person-centred approach and imaging is new to many students. It takes much time and practice to relinquish that which impedes, to acquire a new approach. Learning a new language takes time. Based on self and peer assessment, on-going feedback caringly given, students can see their difficulties and their progress. I hope to illustrate this process.

Nina is back; she has a baby girl, Natasha. Jo and Dawn are away. Jo rang, she's ill.

I suggest another exercise:

Exercise with image 15—Magic Gift Shop

'Close you eyes —— you are walking along a street in a town — you come to a side-street — you've never been in this street before—you walk down the side street—you notice a shop — you look into the shop window — There are all kinds of objects from different parts of the world, different times — you go into the shop — the shopkeeper greets you — says: 'Do look around' — perhaps, as you look, you may be drawn to one object in particular —— Maybe you have noticed one such object. You may want to touch it—have a good look at it —Now the shopkeeper says: 'This is an unusual shop. We don't take money. If you want this object for yourself, you need to exchange it for something of yours — and you are thinking, what you might trade in of yours,

> *leave here, so that you can have the object of your choice—and now it is time for you to leave — you go out of the shop—you're in the little side street, walking back to the main street—now you're back in the street where you began— and when you want, open your eyes, come back to this room, portray whatever aspect of your visit to the shop, in whatever way seems right for you — you have 10 minutes — you have some 3-4 minutes now — finish off now —.'*

The students work in two groups of four—two observers, one client, one counsellor, with 15 minutes from each corner.

We come together, to share. Students are listening/reflecting better, reflecting aspects of the picture—colour, size, position. Now and then they interpret—the client knows this is uncomfortable, she is not being deeply understood.

At this stage not enough 'bridges'—links between the person and the image—are being made, to help the person know what the image says for her.

Nina talks of a room full of rubbish which becomes transformed into a beautiful place, free of conflict. What's that about for her?

The image is trying to speak in its symbolic language; the counsellor, in working creatively, can help the client to break the code.

Wendy wants a vibrating golden ball, giving off light, not of this word (the world of duties), she needs to trade in—let go of—the clutter of her previous marriage—to have space for herself—want versus should.

Rosemary has a treasure box with keyhole and keys—she doesn't know what's in it. Is she to give up a precious ring? The issue: to risk the unknown for the safe and familiar.

For Geraldine, the emerging message is: she knows what she wants.

Marianne wants a bright light, has to give up fear. 'When I give up fear, I get what I want, become enlightened.' The light in the picture fits the word. *See Fig. 21.*

This happens frequently; the *word* of the image sounds like a significant issue for the client: the woman who drew a wishing well; that week she was due for an operation. She was wishing to be well. The woman who drew a setting sun; 'the *sun* is going down and there's nothing I can do about it.' Her mentally handicapped *son* might be going down.

And it is with 'bridges' that the message of the picture becomes known. Once known, you may need to work on that issue. But the picture has done its job—made you aware of some aspect from the unconscious—a hope, a fear—suppressed from your awareness, which needs to be integrated in order that you can move towards your potential.

We have experienced five exercises this term; I ask the students to share what they've discovered about person-centred art therapy for themselves.

Nina: It's very powerful.

Heather: It short-circuits verbal modes.

Geraldine: You can trust what it reveals.

Rosemary: And the picture goes on speaking to me during the week.

Wendy: The problem comes to the fore with each exercise.

With Wendy, each picture brings up the same theme: more time for *her*, less duties. It is not enough to hear, and hear again, the message—her hope, her wish for more space. Will she respond?

Later, Marianne writes:

'...I was drawn to an old-fashioned lamp. I thought of Diogenes with his lamp, 'looking for one honest man' ('woman'). I wanted to give up my uncertainty. The lamp, both a search and an answer—an enlightenment. The grey cloud, lack of faith in me. I want to shine with understanding and love—when I do, the cloud will disappear. I'll have found this honest woman—Me.—Stop holding back Marianne you fool!' *See Fig. 21.*

Comments

Jo is away again—I'm concerned, wondering if there's a 'message behind the message'; is there something she's not saying?

The students arrive each week, like children to a party, with the excited expectation of another art therapy exercise. Me, pulling a rabbit out of a hat; a wondrous and burdensome role; I need to know that sometimes the hat may be empty, and that's O.K. Then I can be Liesl, not a magician.

One swallow doesn't make a summer: Practise is the best way forward.

Students discover—again—the importance of experiential learning. Rogers sees the primary task of the teacher to 'permit the student to learn.' Find out for herself. The person-centred way. Students—as clients—find out for themselves that the person-centred facilitative approach applied to the image enables them to feel deeply understood, fully accepted, enabling them to become more aware, move on, develop, grow. Students see how quickly the theme of the image can emerge. As counsellors, from feedback, they are aware of their progress and their difficulties.

Each week, a magical mystery tour, as unaware material rises from the images, becomes known. Quite awe-inspiring.

Students have further opportunity to facilitate, to give and receive feedback. Wider reflections can be made with previous images—A series can have more potential than a 'one-off'': what is it that keeps coming up? What is required of me in response?

The potential of this guided fantasy can be: 'What I want and what I need to do to get it.'

Students can see where and when such an exercise might be appropriate.

Application

In any situation where personal development is the issue—individual, pairs, groups, in training, in therapy.

Person-centred art therapy can be offered whenever the facilitator intuits that this is the moment to reach right-side of the brain material.

SESSION EIGHTEEN
Person-centred Supervision
Forming of
assessment groups
a Valentine Card

"Nobody on earth can give you either the key or the door to open, except yourself."

Krishnamurti

Purpose

To select assessment groups.
To share work issues.
To experience person-centred supervision.
To practice listening/reflecting.
To use a 'diary' date—Valentine's day—for an art therapy exercise.

Jo is still away, ill.

The first object is for students to select assessment groups. They do so by the same random procedure used for ratifying, this time with the numbers 1-10. Each person pulls a number out of a hat—her number. This is then placed on a rotating grid: she is assessed by the three numbers after her; she assesses the three numbers before her. Noone assessing someone who is assessing her. No overlap. No contamination. Now they know the six people with whom they may want to work in particular, for assessment purposes, both to be assessed, and to assess.

Next: Supervision. Time to share work problems. To begin with, each student describes her work:

Heather is in a psychiatric adolescent unit for 11-17 year olds.

Kim is a teacher, working with two groups of 9 year olds.
Marianne does one-to-one counselling in an alcoholic dependency centre.
Mary is a nurse both on a ward for the terminally ill, and in a community care unit—a day unit.
Dawn is between jobs—has one client.
Rosemary is a voluntary worker in the art therapy department of a psychiatric hospital.
Geraldine is a Relate counsellor, and a counsellor for women with eating disorders.
Nina is an educational social worker, seeing children at a school and at home.
Wendy is a coordinator of a cancer self-help group and has two clients, one-to-one.
Jo—absent—is a photo therapist.
Mary, Marianne, Geraldine, Heather and Kim want to talk about a work issue.

I clarify about person-centred supervision: the purpose is to enable the *person* to find her own solution. So, no advice-giving, problem-solving. We reflect. Not by being told, but by being deeply understood, the person may reach her resolution.

In supervision there may be a case for some information giving.

'I could do with a book on the subject, but don't have one'. Reflecting 'so you don't know of a book you want' may not be appropriate if you do know of a book! But watch the fine dividing line, when it's OK to give information, when not.

Mary begins:
She is setting up an art therapy group, has cleared it with management: Wednesdays from 2-3 pm for six weeks. Membership based on self-selection. It will be a closed group.
The problem: How to arrange the seating.
M: I thought I'd have a big table in the middle and we'd sit

round it. But I want it to be like here—sitting on the floor. But one person is in a wheelchair, the others are elderly. (Group members simply reflect— she hears herself)

M: As I'm speaking, I can see it's OK for us to be sitting round a table.

The issue is: how to adapt and amend that which we do here, to the workplace. Getting into the reality of the client and setting up a structure through the client's eyes, appropriate for the client.

Later, Mary adds: I felt I came to the answer myself—the group helped by reflecting and summarising, by letting me hear myself.

Marianne:

The problem: She works in an agency where clients are required to be sober before they can be seen, where behavioural goal-setting is the model.

M: 'I want to be person-centred in a task-centred model.' Again, as she talks, as members reflect, she says: 'As I hear myself, I think it's perfectly OK for both—I can be person-centred within this structure.'

Geraldine:

Talks about an anorexic patient.

The problem: She wants to be person-centred, but finds it hard to see the client losing weight, when her thinking becomes distorted, her life is in danger. The client's mother is anxious. The client is on an eating programme in hospital. The doctor wants results. The client shares feelings, and uses art therapy to see herself. As Geraldine talks, as she hears herself talk, through the reflecting of group members, she comes to see that her task is to be available to the *client*, in a person-centred way. She's doing OK. Mother's anxiety, the doctor's pressure, are not her problems. Again, she gets there for herself.

Heather:

The problem: A boy in her group produces an image (a colourless dragon) but won't talk about it.

H: 'I'm thrilled when he paints, frustrated when he won't talk.'

Having the mirror held up to her, she gets to a point where she says: 'It's OK to let him do it at his pace. I needed to hear myself say it.'

The issue of conditional acceptance. Wanting the client to be how I want him to be. You can't push the river. The client picks up the unaccepting attitude (she's not pleased when I don't talk), will defend himself further. Letting be—the order of the day.

Kim:

Talks about a boy who painted a house—father is no longer there—and has refused to talk about it any more.

Another boy draws cartoon characters. Kim gets him to associate: 'Are you like the rabbit?' He shuts up.

As she talks, she too sees she must allow the process. The client is not there to accommodate the counsellor.

Here the issue is something about pace: with both boys she made 'bridges' very early on, before enough trust had been established, and the client back-tracked. You need to keep your finger on the pulse of the process, to intuit the appropriate pace. It's a bit like eating: you chew a morsel, swallow it, need a bit of time before you're ready for the next bite. Each person has her own pace. If you stuff food down her, she may throw up.

Sometimes it is therapeutic for a child simply to express in images an issue of worry, fear, trauma; the symbolic process of letting out, onto an image, without words, is a release. On some level the child knows its world, what it's doing, expressing, telling in picture form.

The issues were mainly about adjusting to the reality of the client, and of accepting the client. 'As I hear myself,'—

says Marianne—as others speak Marianne back to her: the proof of good person-centred practice.

Group members saw again the benefit of the person-centred approach; letting the person get there.

There are many settings where this kind of supervision could be used.

Exercise with image 16: A Valentine Card
It is Valentine's Day.
I suggest we each make a card: think of someone important to you—in your present life, from your past, perhaps yourself. Take paper, fold it into a card. On the front, put symbols to represent: 'I appreciate'—pause—now open the card. Draw shapes to symbolise: 'I resent'—pause—Now put images about: 'I demand'—on the back section.'

We share in the group.

Heather and Geraldine found it hard to 'demand'—they have no right.

Wendy feels guilty that she *could* demand!

Marianne's was for her father, who died a year ago. She could remember, appreciate him.

Rosemary's card was to herself—she's fed up being for others.

Most people would give their card to the recipient.

Mary is upset she couldn't make a demand—she will give the card to her boyfriend.

Though this exercise is more about illustrating a 'think', (left-side brain), it is a way of expressing feelings regarding a person and learning about oneself, *and* use of colour, position of symbols—the spontaneous elements—can reveal aspects not known before. Not the sort of card you get in the shops!

Students reported noticing a very positive atmosphere in the group. I mentioned the process of group dynamics: 'Norm—form—storm—perform.' We 'stormed' at the end of last term—now we can perform. No storm, no perform.

Comments

In the supervision session, students could watch each other facilitate, note progress since September. Now, there's some real listening, appropriate reflecting. They're getting the hang of it, and are pleased. How to extend this skill, creatively, to the image world requires further attention.

When students share problems from work in this session they highlight central issues familiar to many, e.g.:

The need to refer to a highway code of 'shoulds' rather than trusting intuition, being flexible;

identifying with the client's material, and the ensuing need for supervision;

the need to be perfect 100% of the time, no matter what;

non-acceptance of the client;

taking the focus away from the client to other personae in the scenario;

Issues of accountability within organisations, and of particular relevance for us;

how it is to be the only one in an institution/group modelling the person-centre approach

And so, together, the students listen, identify, and learn. Geraldine leaves her card behind: what is she not taking with her? I'm puzzled.

I enjoy sitting back, watching the students get there! One of the great pleasures of teaching in this way.

Application

Supervision: In all settings where work is supervised—training, learning, work.

Valentine card: In all settings to do with personal development—counselling, art therapy, Relate counselling, inter-personal skills work, etc.

SESSION NINETEEN
Imaging without a theme

"In imagination, not in perception, lies the substance of experience, while science and reason are but it's chastened form."

Santayana

Purpose

To experience spontaneous imaging, without the 'prop' of a structure.
To work in the group—more practice.
To give/receive feedback.

Jo is back.

Today I want to offer an exercise to engage the imagination with as little structure as possible. No guided fantasy, as in the magic gift shop, to lead one from left-side thought to right-side spontaneous image; no metaphor—animal, rose bush—as an outlet for the image—and whatever subconscious material is thereby projected. No hook for the imagination.

Rather, a means whereby, the thinking quiet, the mind blank, one can let an image come, of itself. Whatever is there, to surface.

Children, the mentally handicapped, those in touch with their creative imaginative aspects, those, in other words, not preoccupied with thought, reason, and judgement, hardly need a device, an exercise, to connect with their image world. It is enough to say: 'Close your eyes—see what image floats up for you.' Or: take paper and paint, and spontaneously draw, whatever comes.'

So today's exercise, in the hope that students are, by now, tapping into their image world more readily, that the rust on the hinges of the gate between left and right side of the brain has been rubbed off, the gate well-oiled, an exercise for more spontaneous imaging.

Exercise with image 17—Circle walk
The students form a circle, turn to the right. They are asked to walk round in a circle, taking regular, rhythmic steps, looking at their feet, thinking of nothing, getting into a meditative quiet mood — a meditative slow walk—and then — as they walk on and on—see if an image comes up...When ready, to stay with the image and to portray it.

For each student, after working on the image, some issue has emerged, some aspect not in the forefront of her awareness, but requiring attention, integration. Symbolic messages from the subconscious making themselves known.

They decide to work as a group, one 'client', talking about her picture; the rest; half 'counsellors', half 'observers', to give feedback. I act as 'observer'.

So:

Jo draws a picture of footsteps leading to 'raw sewage'. 'I need to cross it or go back. I can't go round it—I must go through it.' 'It's life in a nutshell.' See Fig. 22.

The 'counsellors' were reflecting back Jo's words, were reflecting aspects of the picture. They were not making 'bridges'—linking the picture, the issue of going through the sewage, to Jo's life. They seemed to be avoiding the sewage. When a counsellor is unwilling to deal with heavy material—here, going through sewage, could be the shit in Jo's life—she needs to ask herself, perhaps in her own supervision, what this is a bout for *her*—probably some material of her own being avoided, and needing attention. She won't harm the client by such avoidance. Neither will she move her on.

And Kim too: on one page she draws women walking in the circle. She laughs. 'I can smell them.'

On another page, a person behind bars: 'It's a prison

courtyard.' 'I put myself in prison', 'I'm laughing at the dark side of life—I survive using humour.' *See Fig. 23.*

Again, the 'counsellors' leave out the 'heavy' issues, don't get Kim to link the picture and herself, to associate it with the dark side of her life now.

Nina draws a spiral. She is baffled. 'It's mindless, no purpose, just going round and round.' 'There's no beginning, no end.' The 'counsellors' reflect well, ask Nina to connect, associate, make a bridge. She can't/won't.

Sometimes the 'client' doesn't, isn't ready to see the message of the picture. The picture—as against words—keeps; she may, at a later time, have a moment of insight. Or not.

The picture—some aspect of the unaware. Perhaps in the forefront of Nina's awareness are issues with purpose, with structure. Logos. What of the flip side? The 'mind-less' side?

Similarly, Rosemary draws a circle with 'a flowery shape on top.' 'I'm mystified. I half-saw' Her life at present is 'bubbling over, going well.' What of the mystified, half seen aspects, knocking on her door?

Marianne, too, portrayed the picture and, in speaking of it, unselfconsciously, describes herself. She draws a Tai Chi dancer. 'The dancer didn't come out right—is too rigid, not moving enough.' Link to Marianne—yes, she can own this, can go on to say: 'I need to be like the dancer—without shoes—grounded; strong by being soft, and balanced.'

One of the advantages of talking about a picture—rather than simply talking to someone—is that the client loses herself in the picture, becomes more spontaneous, less guarded. It is then that her words are unpremeditated. She is using language as it were, with right side of brain intelligence, releasing moments of existential truth about herself.

So, whilst walking in the circle, an image comes; whilst drawing it, I may not know its meaning. Only when the picture and my words, both, are reflected to me, played back to me, in a way that helps me make a link between the picture and myself, then I can come to know its message. That in itself is not enough. Then the work begins of integrating the revealed message. Marianne wants to be like the dancer. The wish. She may need to work on herself, to actualise the wish.

Comments

It is becoming clear that the counsellor, at her most effective, is creative, is in touch with her 'right-side brain'; is spontaneous, works alongside the client, in the moment. The less she thinks, judges, worries, the more she trusts herself to the moment, her journey alongside her client may be an exciting one towards growth. Both the client's, and her own, as she frees herself from the waterwings of thought, and connects with her intuition, imagination, inspiration. The magical mystery tour of self-discovery. Being enabled to become more whole in a non-judgemental client-centred way. If that is all she achieves during the year, to re-discover, re -connect with her feminine principle of knowing—be it as client or counsellor—it is more than enough. The certificate, a fringe benefit needed only in the 'real' world, where such pieces of paper open doors. The *real* gift is the self-discovered learning about the self.

Another way to work with free imaging is to suggest that the 'client' take paper and draw/paint quite spontaneously whatever comes. No plan, developing the process 'on the hoof'.

Recently, over a period of days, I made a series of spontaneous pictures—tearing out bits, burning bits, covering bits up—which all fitted; I was creating a symbolic process of deep significance which I need to face, to own, to be.

So, once the creative process flows, no need for exercises, 'hooks': just produce the image, and welcome its message, for it is a gift from your subconscious which you need to receive at this very time. It makes me wonder how much of a potential therapy component there is in the art on view in art galleries.

I'm aware, often, that images release much heavy material. Whatever the students do with it, wherever they take it, a collection of heavy vibes is released in the room, week after week. How do I deal with them, not to get overwhelmed by them myself. A ritual of ventilating the room, letting in fresh air, is my non-verbal way of preparing the room—and me—for the next session.

Application

In any training/learning/therapy situation to encourage connecting with right-side intelligence.

The reader can be as flexible and creative in applying any of these exercises.

SESSION TWENTY
Fairytale

"Une fée est cachée en tout ce que tu vois."

Victor Hugo

Purpose

To encounter the world of myth and fairytale, allegorical stories of the inner life.

To experience for oneself an art therapy exercise in a group; the possibility of using the images produced by others for one's own projections.

To practice person-centred facilitating.

To look at emerging issues of personal boundaries, rights, risk-taking, trust, and inter-personal interaction.

Jo has rung; she is ill.
    Geraldine is away again.
    Today I want to shift the focus in two ways:
    a) that the image is drawn on a shared piece of paper;
    b) that the theme is in the realm of myth, fairytale.
    More of the purpose later.

Exercise with image 18—'Once upon a time'

The students sit in two rows of five, each row has a long sheet of paper before it. I say:

'Draw a story which begins with: "Once upon a time." A story about some creature, some being of your choice. Start your story on the part of the paper in front of you, and then, see where else you might want to go with your story.'

They draw. They stay put. Only Heather gets up and draws a little 'person' along the whole length of the paper, along the other student's images.

    They sit back. Stop.

We discuss: What did they make of the 'instruction'?

Dawn: I wanted to spread out, but I mustn't take up too much space.

L: Is that right, do you have that belief about you?'

Dawn: Yes.

Marianne: I heard—but I assumed we'd sit back and compare our pictures. (*Never work on assumptions, always check out assumptions.*)

Heather: I wanted to continue my story on the whole space; I thought: this is fun. Then I saw I was the only one. I sat down in my place each time I'd drawn my little figure on someone else's space. I became tentative. What if I'll look foolish?

L: Is that right?—you know what you want to do, you do it, and when you see you're the only one, you're afraid you'll be seen as stupid, you hold back.

H: Yes.

Mary: I wanted to go over to my right—but time was up (*I had said: 'You have 20 minutes,'—and, later: 'You have 10 minutes.'*)

L: So you decide to risk it when time's up.

Here we see how a small film clip of a student's behaviour, when described without self-consciousness, and when reflected back, can bring to her awareness a belief of herself to herself—the behaviour illustrating that belief.

Kim: I wanted to go across—I thought she'd be cross.

The issue about boundaries, about the right to more space, about stopping yourself even when the instructions give you permission to go into other territory.

The issue about safety versus risk—and what you forego by playing it safe.

In this case, the creative opportunity to project your story onto the images put down by others—the freedom of the spontaneous flow, in a wider setting.

I have offered this exercise with groups, where each member moved along freely, continuing her story on the images already created by others, each seeing the same image differently, for her own unique purpose. So here, in this group, we have a series of separate images (except Heather) on one paper—as if they'd worked separately. Perhaps, paradoxically, we learn more about ourselves from that which we didn't do, from that which we didn't risk, from that which we found difficult, than from the easy, manageable, unproblematic.

They 'debrief' in their two groups of five—one client, one or two counsellors, one—or two—observers.

The second strand to the exercise, to engage the person in the world of fairytale, myth; the opportunity to tell some aspect of yourself in a different, more magical frame of reference, leading to insights quite unavailable to the realm of mere thoughts. Mythological characters, archetypal, symbolic aspects of the self, making themselves known.

Marianne saw her story as that of 'Jack and Jill', the bit that drew her: 'Jack fell down,' her own falls, on the way up her hill.

Nina drew a small dot, becoming a chrysalis, becoming a beautiful butterfly. The process of 'growth, development, transformation '—both the wish for the baby she has just had, and for herself. *See Fig. 24 (Colour).*

Dawn drew a person with three heads—happy, strong and depressed—how to maintain the balance. The body was herself: 'strong, together, powerful and beautiful in my own right,' the tree with its branches, for her to lie under, rest, refresh herself, give herself the balance between work and rest. *See Fig. 25 (Colour).*

Students talked of the issue of risk:

Kim: 'I take a risk with my picture—what will I find, will I be ready for something unexpected?'

It is my belief that the client sees what she is ready to see.

Nina: That's why I like the person-centred approach; 'you stay with the client, don't push her to areas she's not ready to know.' Exactly.

Heather went on to talk of the risk of changing as a result

of self-awareness; others perceive you changing, and may not like the changing you. She reports how different she is at work now—not everyone too pleased.

Rosemary reports how she stood up to a teacher at a parent's meeting last night. wanting her son to be present at a discussion which was, after all, about him. She was heard—the son joined in. A 'first' for Rosemary.

I mentioned the sequence of:

—knowing—owning—acting—in the business of self-discovery.

Applied to art therapy, the image may reveal a truth about yourself which you need to know. 'Knowing'. Now you know. That's not all of it. You need to move on to 'owning' the feelings around the issue, in order to release yourself, and 'act'—move to a new more helpful behaviour.

Comments

The realm of myth and fairytale is powerful; to transpose your story, or part of it—an event, a sequence, which was difficult, perhaps in terms of 'once upon a time', can bring quite amazing insights. It is as if we cross the frontier of reality to a land of far richer potential, where we may find treasures much needed on our road to self-awareness.

Overall, students have come a long way since September, in listening with more attention. Now and then there is an interpretation, when both the client and the counsellor are aware of the 'hiccup', perceive it is intrusive and unhelpful. Some students still focus predominantly on words. They need to take regard more of the image, and all its aspects. They need to make more 'bridges' connecting the picture and the person, allowing the images to speak. The pace of some students is too fast; they do not allow the 'client' sufficient time to digest an intervention. They are more 'counsellor-centred', busy with their own process, their need to point out the next bit, rather than being 'client-centred', tuning in to the pace of the client. I need to repeat these by now familiar observations from the sidelines, to show that there is progress, and that much more practice is needed. Patience!

When students operate from 'shoulds' (what should I say?) from thoughts, from 'left-side of the brain', they stop themselves from taking off, from going along with the client, spontaneously, creatively, from moment to moment. Both counsellor and client needing to be in touch with their creative existential aspect, to actualise the potential of the emerging work. Students need to listen more intuitively, know, in their gut, what needs attention—be it phrase, image, an earlier connection; making links between any of these—whatever is THERE. An exciting business. I am pointing the way ahead. They're on the right road, having travelled a good way already.

And I'm left wondering about Geraldine's absence. Her reason: a shattered windscreen as she was about to leave her house. What's that symbolism, in her myth?

Application

The group picture: Any group working together.

Myth: can be applied more widely and fruitfully in personal development.

THE DAY
Individual and group work with images.
Themes: (a) Mother, (b) an Island

"It is never too late, sometimes it is too soon."
Buddhist saying

Daughter am I in my mother's house,
But mistress in my own.
The gates are mine to open,
As the gates are mine to close,
And I abide by my Mother's House.
Our Lady of the Snows —Rudyard Kipling

Purpose

To deal with the loss of a group member.

To experience a group art therapy exercise in order to see both personal and inter-personal issues.

To learn about our group dynamic from the image.

To explore the theme 'mother' with an image.

Ever more practice.

To experience working for a longer period with an image.

We gather.

Geraldine—who has missed the last two sessions—says she is leaving the group. (I am amazed, surprised). She tells me that once I made a link between her own issue of overeating when anxious, needing to hide her body and work with anorexics. On another occasion, she says, I gave her feedback, that she had avoided the anger of the client. She perceived both these comments as put downs. She, an accredited Relate counsellor, no long rescues, avoids; has done her work on her own bulemia. She feels unvalued and has come to say goodbye. She wants my response.

I am still stunned:—I say that there'd been no congruent message from Geraldine, no clue, no warning. A bombshell. Geraldine, so actively, enthusiastically involved throughout. My gut tells me this blaming does not belong to me: I feel I'd given her level feedback. By the time it reached her, she seems to have transposed it to a criticism, can't allow it in, hear it. I believe she is throwing out the baby with the bathwater; what about all my warm affirming positive feedback, my acknowledgment of the amazing magical material which kept surfacing for her in her images. I feel really sad—I'm tearful—at her news, at her leaving, the suddenness. I value her, feel warmly for her, saw her as an important actively involved member of the group. I appreciate that she was able to come and say goodbye; that took courage. Other group members express surprise and regret, give positive feedback. Geraldine walks to the door—we go up to her to embrace her. She leaves.

We share our feelings of sadness, anger, surprise, shock, I suggest we focus on 'I' statements rather than 'gossip'— about the absent Geraldine. 'Talking about' someone changes nothing.

Again, we see how 'process' needs attention, whatever 'content' had been planned for the day.

We are aware, too, that Jo is away for the fourth time. She rings each time, says she is ill, or now very busy with her work, hopes to come next time. Will she? Has she left?

Exercise image 19—Group Island
The intention had been for an individual art therapy exercise in the morning.
I suggest we do a group exercise now, so as:

(a) to have the opportunity to express how we feel now, in the wake of Geraldine's leaving, as a group.

(b) to share any personal material which might emerge;

(c) to facilitate;

(d) to learn about our group dynamic—the inter-personal aspect—from the image.
> We tape up a large sheet of paper. I draw the outline of an island. I say: 'This is your island. You are living on this island together.' Everyone gets busy; after 20 minutes of drawing, we stop. We agree that group members would talk about their individual imput, then we would look at what the picture says about the group dynamic.

It soon emerges that the individual pictures contained strategies in the wake of loss and change:

Mary draws a large tree in the middle of the island, with fruit for all, and a sun to shine on all: she wants to make everything sunny for everyone, after a loss—she needs to compensate—repeating a familiar strategy to do with the death of her parents.

Marianne gets busy being very practical—building a shelter, planning etc.—she is full of emotion and this activity avoids them: her way of coping with loss.

Heather needs to be on her own—at sea, in a cave, and on top of a tree—she feels overwhelmed and needs to separate, digest, allow in, before being able to reconnect with others. A familiar pattern for her in the wake of separation.

Other personal issues emerged too:

Rosemary needs to risk going to an unknown island, offshore. She gives herself a boat too small for the purpose—sabotages herself, doesn't let herself have what she needs in order to do what she wants.

Dawn—may have M.E.—needs to sit quietly on the beach, after too much activity. The recurring 'wish'.

Kim draws a Venus arising from the sea who turns into a Christ—a female Christ on the cross holding a coconut—she needs to become herself—and, like Asher Lev—defies her family's disapproval. She needs nourishment in this process. *See Fig. 26.*

Wendy—first brings herself, then gives love and nourishment to others.

Students feel relieved that, with the language of art, they could spontaneously express their reaction to Geraldine's going. We feel we have moved on, are more available to our programme.

Now, a look—literally—at the group dynamic:

We look at each person's image in a different way: what does it say about her role in the group:

> Heather brings positive energy, power, reliability, and commitment.
>
> Kim risks sharing her pain, confronts.
>
> Wendy quests for her personal autonomy.
>
> Mary feels for others—'floods'—gives too much.
>
> Rosemary confronts—says what's difficult.
>
> Dawn needs to be low/vulnerable.
>
> Marianne is strong being gentle.
>
> And I—I gave the island—the structure.

In any group, if members are unaware of the quality each individual manifests in the group, then it could be that there is a collusion to off-load, each member made to carry that aspect for the rest of the group; unable to integrate other aspects of the self. For example: Dawn could (if the group is unaware) carry vulnerability. Then others can be strong. She can't be in touch with her strength. Kim could become the one to share pain—has little chance to be frivolous, joyful. And the opposite of this formula: the others can't get in touch with their vulnerability, their pain—whilst they let Dawn and Kim do it for them. Once aware of this prospect, the danger is reduced; it is possible for each to be more fully, awarely, all of herself.

Such unaware collusion often occurs in couples, the partners drawn to one another, so that, say, the practical, well-organised one chooses the opposite—a dreamer, per-

181

haps. The dreamer lets the partner be practical, can't connect with her own practical facet—and vice versa.

In families, too, members can, unawarely, carry certain aspects for the whole family: the sick one, the deviant, the coper, the dustbin, etc. As in teams, staff groups, committees, any group.

Here we are, learning about our group dynamic, illustrated vividly on the picture, the dynamic projected onto the island.

An art therapy exercise such as today's 'island', when used in groups—whether a family, a team, a management group, members of a ward, household, home, etc—can disclose, very accurately, the group dynamic, the way individual members behave in and for the group: words can conceal, avoid. Images are a true reflection, and when explored safely, in the person-centred way, will make available valuable insights to members of the group, leading to the possibility of more aware responsible behaviour and inter-relatedness in the future.

After a shared lunch, we decide on an exercise to focus on the individual. We think we've attended to the process regarding Geraldine sufficiently, for now, to move on.

Exercise with Image 20: Mother
We have the whole afternoon. Students decide to work in threes. They will have longer to work with the image, discover what this entails.
The students close their eyes, relax. I suggest they image around one word: 'Mother'.
We work with the resulting pictures:

Rosemary's image came—
'I wanted to push it away. I had hoped for something nicer'—and later she says about the image of her mother (an insect):
'I faithfully reproduced it.'
She wanted a nicer mother—and she is faithfully reproducing mother. How? She could express much about

the mother—'a hovering insect—with a sting in her tail—you'd never know when she'd land—unpredictable.'

And how does Rosemary 'faithfully reproduce' any of this? Perhaps in herself? The picture leads to further exploration. *See Fig. 27.*

Feedback:

Wendy, as counsellor, does not listen to Rosemary sufficiently, is busy with her own process of thinking of the next intervention. Counsellor-centred. She won't harm. Neither will she be of full effect in this way.

Listening is improving all the time. Now: the need to be more flexible, spontaneous, hear and see the significant issues, move creatively from moment to moment, with the client. I need to speak this aim repeatedly, to keep it before the students, as a focus.

Students had longer to draw, and to talk about the picture.

Dawn: I liked more time to draw—more time for me. There was too much time to talk about it.

Marianne: I enjoyed the freedom, the permission, to take up more time.

Mary: I'm not used to longer time. I prefer the familiar.

After work on 'mother', with five minutes left, Kim wants to discuss a work issue. After five minutes, I say I am too tired to pay full attention now. Others agree.

The issue might be: how do I ask for help at a time when I'm likely to get it? Or not. 'Mother'—a big issue for Kim—so let's talk about work—when we're all tired, at the end of a full day.

What a day! The two themes—'loss and change', and 'mother', probably at the top of the table of issues brought to counselling.

Heather: Loss and mother have exhausted me. (Quite so!)

We agree we have navigated well through the day. The 'island' goes up on the wall. We feel close.

Rosemary: 'With each loss the group is stronger.' A paradox.

I give a 'health warning', you may have tapped into some deep material during the day, to do with such big themes, and the process may continue; you may have insights, make connections, dream a big dream.

Take care of yourself!

Marianne writes:

'Mother' *See Fig. 28.*

The pink; the warmth, the good feelings I felt with mother when young. Me grown up, pulling away, why the chains? I rarely see my mother, she isn't particularly demanding in an outward sense.

But the chains are there. Chains of guilt because I no longer feel good when I'm with her. The familiar ties are there but I don't relish seeing her, it's a duty and a *burden* as is shown in the picture.

I really drew the picture without much thought, it just evolved. And, when I looked at it recently I was amazed to see that the shape which held mother and me was the shape of a foetus! I hadn't realised that at all. The chain, the umbilical cord!

This exercise evoked tremendous stirrings of a variety of emotions, most of which I did not feel comfortable with, the lost security, the struggle, guilt, love, hate.

Somebody (a client) said to me recently "there's worse things than not being cuddled I suppose", referring to her childhood.

I contemplated this remark, I had lots of cuddles as a child. I wondered if not being listened to was one of the worse things.'

Because of the image, Marianne could get further, later.

Comments

I regret Geraldine's leaving; she gave much, and had much to gain.

I recall being amazed and enthusiastic about the recurring magical aspects of her images, and Geraldine saying she didn't see them that way, was nervous and apprehensive of the magic. I was not open to her reality.

I'm pleased I offered the group island exercise in the wake of this loss—symbolically contacting individual feelings around loss, in a group.

The 'mother' exercise: mother—one of the main issues in therapy. By offering the possibility of non-verbal knowing, a far deeper level of awareness is possible.

Application

The group exercise: In any group, team, management, committee, working together, where the understanding of the group dynamic is a valuable means to optimum functioning.

Mother in therapy, counselling—for anyone needing to explore this theme. In short: for all!

SESSION TWENTY-ONE
(1) Using an existing image (Tarot cards), a taster of gestalt
(2) Gestalt exercises

"If you want to draw a bird you must become a bird."

Hokusai

Purpose

To give a taster of gestalt.
To experience use of an existing image.

We note that Jo is away again. We decide to contact her, check out her intentions.

Exercise with image 21—Projecting onto an existing image: Tarot

I explain that I am using the cards just for their pictures, we are not working with them in a 'Tarot' way.

I spread out a pack of Tarot cards on the floor. The students are asked to look at them and see which card they are drawn to quite spontaneously, to represent the client in themselves.

They select. They go into pairs. They take turns—four minutes each way—to talk, not about the person on the card, but as the person on the card, to become that person.

I demonstrate: 'I am little. I want to play out here. Let this grown-up here go into the house and deal with the work—I want some fun.'

When they have done this, they choose a card symbolising the 'counsellor' in themselves. Again, in pairs, they speak, becoming the person of the card.

Then they place the two cards side by side. Again, in pairs, they take five minute turns to have a dialogue between the two cards, between 'client' and 'counsellor'. Not about them, but engaging, creatively and imaginatively in a conversation, now being 'client', now being 'counsellor'.

We have feedback;

For some, the conversation was very real; they reached new awarenesses, even resolved a problem.

Now I say that this was a 'sample' of 'gestalt'. I like an experiential component first, before the theory. Now the students already know what I mean when I explain the theory—they've tried it out for size.

Gestalt is about being aware, about bringing that which is in the background of awareness to the foreground, to bring about integration. It is about 'coming out of your head and into your senses.' Not thinking, explaining, but open to the moment, to spontaneous knowing by way of feeling, sensing, being—very similar to the existential creative process.

In the exercise we separated out two aspects of the self, to engage in a dialogue. This dramatic way brings about an immediacy, a clarity. When we talk 'about', a distancing occurs and, with it, less opportunity to make connections with oneself.

The exercise showed:

a) Using the tarot cards, we did not need to draw, but projected onto an existing image. The spontaneous choice proving most apt and accurate.

Using picture postcards, pictures from magazines, are other options. Each exercise we do here can be flexibly creatively adjusted depending on the setting, the purpose. There is no highway code: spontaneously, creatively, invent, devise for yourself, for the now.

b) That there is a wise person, a 'counsellor' within each of us; whenever we have a problem, we could engage in such a dialogue, get in touch with our wise self and perhaps come to know the solution.

This 'separating' of two aspects—or two people—is referred to in gestalt as 'cushion' or 'chair' work: sitting on one cushion, becoming one aspect or person and, on the other, becoming another aspect or person; engaging in a dialogue, moving back and forth, so real, so in the moment, with potential for insights.

Exercise 27—Symptom dialogue
I say something like:
'Close your eyes—think of some symptom that bothers you repeatedly—where in your body is this symptom—what do you feel in these parts of your body—Now become this symptom—what are you like—what do you do to this person — Now talk to this person—tell her how you make her feel—what are you saying to her—how do you say? —Now become yourself again and talk back to the symptom—what do you say? — Now become the symptom again—tell this person what you do for her—how are you useful to her—what do you help her avoid — Now become yourself again—what do you answer now?—Take a little while absorbing this experience.
Now open you eyes. Share your experience in the first person, present tense, to own the immediacy, bring it to the now.'

In feedback, Dawn, who may have M.E., recognises that her symptom helps her avoid fulfilling other people's expectations. She is determined to go *her* way more, without being ill.

Marianne sees that she must not avoid but face the pain.

Rosemary is surprised by the viciousness of her symptom wanting to stop her (trapped nerve in neck).

A symptom can have valuable messages for us. In the alliance of head, feelings and body, it can happen that head does not want to acknowledge feelings. So feelings ask body to produce a symptom, perhaps head will listen then. If not, the body might send a stronger symptom. We ignore it and its message at our peril.

There is much evidence that over 85% of symptoms have a psychosomatic component. If only doctors were trained to work with symptoms more holistically, rather than just eliminating the symptom—and its message.

Imaging can be used very effectively with symptoms. Either, after the symptom dialogue, the client can be invited to draw an image of the experience, and continue the dialogue, or the client can be asked to allow an image of the symptom to emerge, and to draw/paint it. Then work can be done with the image as a potent focus. This can lead to the expression of feelings for which the symptom was a deputy. Once expressed, the symptom itself can diminish, disappear.

Exercise 28: Parent or Partner dialogue
They are in pairs. One partner becomes either her own parent or her partner, and talks to the other person about herself.

So: Dawn *becomes* her mother, and talks about her daughter Dawn to her listener:

In feedback, Dawn was surprised about aspects she hadn't known before.

Wendy says: 'It's amazing what you say when you don't think.' Precisely. This is the point of gestalt. Awareness through not thinking. Gestalt aims to frustrate thinking.

Exercise 29: Eating a biscuit
I hand out biscuits. I say: 'As you eat this biscuit, of what are you aware—without thinking, analysing.'
Feedback:
I tasted the salt.
I heard the sound in my mouth, the sound of others crunching,
Felt the sun on my face.
The smell of the biscuit,
Felt the food going round my mouth.

So often, when we think, we are out of touch with our senses, touch, sight, smell, taste, sound. Perhaps we look, and then think to help us label, understand, intellectualise.

So often, when we eat, we are unaware of the process. Here we just held the awareness for a few minutes, while eating, and so much sensing, noticing emerged, enriching the experience.

Being, rather than doing.

This lead us to cordless phones, to walkmans, how they symbolise ever less being, ever more doing in our culture, filling every moment. Yet it is so important to balance periods of 'doing' with times of stillness, meditation, reflection. Being. The experience such as eating a biscuit with awareness, to be taken away from the course, into our daily lives.

Today was a mere taster of gestalt. To train in this way takes years. Next week we will see how this approach can be used dramatically and effectively with art work.

Rosemary adds: In the exercise with the tarot cards, I pick up the card 'Magician'. It has my favourite colours. The second card, the Ace of Wands, again I am attracted by the magical content. The dialogue is: 'I want to be able to do magic. I want to use my wand to help others.' What makes you think you have the power? 'I know I have the power. Now I want to use it.'

'In the parent dialogue, when I was my mother, I was very critical of me, Rosemary. All the negative stuff came out, as well as the boasting of my intellectual achievements which she values in me, rather than the qualities I value in me, such as creativity, spontaneity and emotional expression. Now I need the courage to check out these perceptions with her. In the symptom dialogue I was startled to discover that my symptom called me a bitch, gloated that it prevented me from doing things I want to do.

In eating the cracker, noticing, tasting, sensing, I made the resolve, as a result, to try to eat slower in future and enjoy.'

Comments

I want to introduce a slight shift: how to project inner material onto an existing image. Today I use Tarot cards. Also, I want to give a taster of Gestalt with the image—rather than talking about aspects of the image, to *become* them, thus experiencing more immediacy. Gestalt, like the person-centred approach, stays with the client, does not lead, interpret. The mode of facilitating is more directive—the facilitator telling the person: *be* the little girl, *be* the pain in your back—or whatever; the direction based on the client's material, not the counsellor's. A more dramatic existential approach, aiming, like imaging, to get the client from the thinking, left side brain to the sensing right side. And therefore it lends itself readily to use with images, as we shall see next week.

I wonder about Jo: has she left without being explicit?

Her pictures so powerful, issues of freedom/oppression, pain/joy, life/death. I need to remind myself this is a training—not a therapy—group; not all such emerging material can be dealt with here; I need to realise that I can't facilitate all such material, and accept the boundaries of my role. Absence also makes me aware of my need to be present: so far, over the years, I've not missed a session. A deep-down anxiety: what if I do?

Application

To incorporate experiencing, sensing.

Tarot: For any setting where problem-solving is relevant.

Symptom dialogue: For anyone working with symptoms: cancer, AIDS, the terminally ill, the addicted, the abused.

Parent/Partner dialogue: In counselling, therapy—any setting where the issue of relating needs to be addressed.

Eating a biscuit: Whenever it is helpful to balance analysing and sensing.

SESSION TWENTY-TWO
Art Therapy and Gestalt—
Exercise with image: Motorbike

"The dream (image) is a message of yourself to yourself, to whatever part of you is listening."

Fritz Perls

Purpose

To bring the Gestalt way of facilitating to an art therapy exercise. To practice.

Jo has notified us she is not coming back, has too much work at present. We decide to write, ask her to join us, so that we can say goodbye, at the beginning or end of the next session.

We share our feelings about Jo and her leaving; this, our fourth loss.

We do an art therapy exercise and will see how Gestalt can be applied to the art work.

Exercise with image 22—a guided fantasy: Motorcycle
'Close you eyes—relax—now imagine that you are a motorcycle...what kind of a motorcycle are you...where do you spend most of your time...where is your home...how do you feel as a motorcycle...?
Now start up and go somewhere...how do you get started...what are your surroundings like...where are you going...?
Look back now—is someone riding you...how do you feel towards your rider—take a little longer getting in touch with all the details of your existence as a motorbike...Now open your eyes —portray your experience as a motorbike.'
The students draw for some 10 minutes.

B.—a past student—has drawn a bike only:
 'Be the motorbike.'

'I'm going along very fast; working well.'
'Be the pedal.'
'I get the bike going—it can't manage without me and my hard work.'
'What's this?'
'The accelerator.'
'Be the accelerator.,
'I get up speed. Without me the bike is slow. Ah, but without me you wouldn't even get started.'
'Who are you now?'
'The pedal. Here. In the middle...'
'And what's this?' (a protrusion at the back of the bike)
'I'm the fantastic bit—not like the rest of me—not useful—words can't describe how fantastic I am.'
'At the back—not useful—fantastic, beyond words to describe...'
B. laughs in recognition. We all laugh. No need to say more! *See Fig. 29.*

Working with different components in the picture, like a director with a cast—a little psycho-drama unfolding from the shapes on the paper, as the client identifies with, becomes each component, hearing herself own the different attributes, as a dialogue develops between the members of the 'cast', the impact can be very immediate and powerful. No 'bridges' needed. B. knew what the 'fantastic' bit of her was! Unlike the tentative approach of the person-centred counsellor, the gestaltist orders: BE the pedal. No vague would-you-like-to-be suggestions, where a 'no' is possible. In that sense, Gestalt is more directive, and also non-directive, for the gestaltist only works with the material given by the client. The belief is person-centred, the interventions are directive.

Missing aspects are brought in:
Rosemary:
Dawn: Be the road.
Rosemary: I'm a bendy road, leading from town to the country, to the sea, I'm a bit rigid and too confined.
Dawn: Be the missing bike.

Rosemary: 'I'm off the page. On a curb in the town I'm looking at ways to get to the sea. I can leave the road and find more interesting paths in the hills.' *See Fig. 30.*

Any thinking, intellectualising, must be frustrated.

Nina: Be the bike.

Marianne: I'm powerful—I can go anywhere, do what I like. Nobody is over me. I have my space. I can do what I like.

Nina: Be the lights.

Marianne: I show the way. I focus on certain things. I show the bike it where it can go, and where not.

The dialogue—similar to wider reflections—can be productive.

Heather—as the bike—:

I'm a powerful old bike. I'm parked across the drive. I live in this shed.

Rosemary: Be the shed.

Heather: There are a lot of things in me—I'm cluttered.

Rosemary: Be the bike—tell the shed how is it for you in the cluttered shed.

Heather: I travel around all day, carrying children about. When I get home I want some space.

Giving yourself up to imagination, to fantasy, freeing yourself from logic, anything is possible. As the client IS each component, each symbolic aspect of herself, lives each bit—rather than talking about, once removed—she OWNS, she hears her words, and she can make important connections.

Some students take to this model easily, some less so. Another option. Another road leading to Rome.

Comments

About Jo's leaving: I'm sad, I'll miss her honest sharing, lively input. Jo, who was the trigger for me to write. Now she's left us to it.

Much later, after the end of the course, Jo and I meet. She tells me, yes, she was busy. But also, very vulnerable and sad; her sister had died after Xmas. She could not share this. When working in threes, feeling vulnerable, she perceived feedback as critical, saw herself as de-skilled. The threesome echoed for her times as a child, with her parents, when she was criticised, felt vulnerable. She couldn't take it and—as then—left.

Four students have now left; the largest number to have left *any* group. And this, the group of the book! (A bit of me whispers: what will people think?) Maybe four group members had to leave so that the remaining group can function in a more trusting, resourceful, creative way. And indeed, the 'survivors' have had greater opportunity for learning than 'easier' groups. There have been groups where the developmental process of 'norm, form, storm, perform' has not reached 'storm', has not, therefore, reached its full potential of performing. This group, for sure, in going through each storm, went on to perform. The paradox, yet again.

I need to accept that students have a right to stay, and to leave. I need to stow away an old tape about 'what did I do wrong, it must be my fault.' They continue on their path, I on mine.

The exercise—as some previous guided fantasies—is a gestalt exercise. The fantasy can be explored just verbally. However, I find the added component, of drawing the fantasy, of making it visible, gives much additional potential: size, position, colour of the different components, what has been left out, as well as the spontaneous words used to describe the fantasy—all possible signposts to awareness.

The examples show the use of the gestalt mode of facilitating. Sometimes it is fruitful to be less purist, more flexible: to make 'bridges'.

So, with Rosemary:

'I'm a bendy road...a bit rigid and too confined.'

Bendy road—rigid, confined; can you associate with this road?

...'I'm the missing bike, off the page...'

The missing bike off the page; what might that be about for you?

So, weaving in the Gestalt mode with the image and the person-centred approach can be a creative way of facilitating.

I am indebted to John Stevens. I have adapted some of the ideas from his book: 'Awareness' for use with art. Today's exercise was such an adaptation.

Application

In any setting where the purpose is to shift from thinking to sensing.

SESSION TWENTY-THREE
Art Exercise in small groups— Draw a house

"I can write all about non-verbal art experience but you won't know the reality of what you can experience with art unless you use the material in your own way and for yourself."

Janie Rhyne

Purpose

To use an art therapy exercise in order to work on the inter-personal aspect.
To practice—note areas of improvement, areas of difficulty.
To offer an appropriate exercise at the end of term—a gift sharing.

Jo couldn't come this week, suggests June 6. We want to ask her to come sooner—by June 6 we'll be busy with assessment.

I mention that during the holiday, students could be writing up 'portfolios'—their gathered evidence of all the aspects in their personal contracts.

I remind students that they have agreed to hand in their portfolios on the third week of next term.

Students comment and question, to clarify, to share feelings.

I want to offer an exercise which shows the inter-personal element.

Exercise with image 23—Draw a house: in small groups

The students form three groups. Each group has one sheet of paper, each group member picks a pen, marker—the colour different to the colour of the others in her group. This is so that individual marks are identifiable. The task is: Now, without talking, draw a house together.
After some ten minutes, they stop. We debrief as follows:

One group are 'clients', one group are 'counsellors', one group 'observers'. We rotate till each group has worked on its picture.

Some examples:
   Dawn draws two round windows.

   Facilitator: You've drawn a round window.

   Dawn: Yes, I want a round window today.

   H: Does that speak to you, round window?

   Dawn: Yes, I like to offer a different perspective, let in the light on something different.

   R: And also, you drew a square window after Wendy drew a square window.

   Dawn: Yes, I like to follow on, to complement.

   M: Can you associate with that behaviour in a relationship? (*Bridge*)

   Dawn: Yes. I like to value what the other says and does.

   K: So you like to respect the other, and offer your own, sometimes different perspective. Both. (*Wider reflection*)

   Dawn: Yes. *See Fig. 31. (Colour)*

Again we see how, when we draw spontaneously, without thought, some microcosmic truth of us emerges. In this exercise: how I can be with others.

Marianne says to the people in her group: *'What paper shall we have?'*

   H: You ask the others what they want.

   M: Yes.

   K: Does that ring bells for you?

   M: Yes. I like other people's good opinion of me.

   H: To the exclusion of asking yourself what paper you want?

   M: Yes.

Marianne takes a blue crayon. Mary, too, takes a blue crayon. Marianne puts back her blue, picks a purple crayon.

   L: What's that procedure about?

   M: Giving others more importance than me.

More of the same.

Here we see how every bit of the process—not just the end product—can be of significance, is worth reflecting.

Rosemary draws a little shed to the side of the house—

'an extra little piece'—the house is too regular.'

'I need space, to be myself within a relationship where I'm watchful not to take over.' *On the island she needed a little island for herself—wider reflection. See Fig. 31. (Colour)*

Exercise 30—Shared end of term summary
As it is the last session of the term, we do an 'end of term report'. In pairs, they share:
What I've discovered about person-centred art therapy.
What I've discovered about me.
What I've discovered about me in the group.

They share. Here, some snippets:

Amazing insights from the images.

The respectful element of the person-centred approach.

Feeling safe and trusting with the person-centred approach.

The difficulty of working through the loss of four group members.

When unable to share feelings, going home unfinished.

Anxiety about writing the portfolios—will I have enough, be good enough.

Initially, coming for the certificate, and now realising there's much else to gain besides—discoveries about the self, opportunities to change, and the risk entailed in changing.

As a family, left by four close relatives, we experienced the most familiar trauma brought to therapy, about loss, abandonment and change.

Heather speculates: maybe they had to leave so that we might be close, trusting, and work creatively together.

Exercise with image 10—Gifts (viz. p.105)
As an end-of-term exercise, and one we missed at the end of last term, because process took precedence—
We sit in a circle, each with a paper before us. We put our name on our sheet, and pass it to the person on the left. (Described on p.107. Now we do it) I repeat:
Look at the name on the paper before you. Think of that person, how you know her, and give her a symbolic gift—something you believe she'd need, like, in view of your perception of her. A gift.
The paper is passed round, till it returns to the owner, containing a gift from each group member. The recipient, too, can give herself a gift.
Each person points to each of her gifts, so that the donor can say something about it.

There is much warmth and closeness in the group—a very different ending to that of last term. Everyone has expressed what needed expressing. We can finish.

Comments

Drawing a house together is a lovely exercise with couples, families, small groups, staff groups, teams, management, revealing much about the way the people concerned relate. When I work with a couple, I might use this exercise—or one similar—in the first session, as a basis for our contract.

Because each person uses a different colour, it is clear to see who contributed what to the picture; who keeps to her space, who dominates, who initiates, who follows—and how others in the group respond. The picture of the house, an externalised projection of how the participants relate here, and in other settings.

The exercise can be offered in a more abstract way by suggesting the participants have a conversation, a dialogue (no words to be used) on paper. Similar issues surface: who starts, who follows etc etc.

There it is, in colour, before your eyes. Produced, spontaneously, without premeditation, judgement, thought—thus an accurate microcosmic film clip of the interactions of those concerned. If reflected, per se, without interpretation, much can be revealed and learned.

The gift-sharing exercise enables people to show how empathic and aware they are (or not) of others. An opportunity to care, affirm, show appreciation and warmth. I remember offering this exercise to kids at an off-site centre of a school: so-called 'tough' kids, who didn't verbalise tenderness, were able, with images, to show how caring, gentle and perceptive they could be. It is a good exercise for endings, celebrations. At a deeper level, it can reveal much about projections—what do the gifts I give say about *me*; am I giving aspects of me to others, how in touch or out of touch am I with others, how is it to express level positive regard.

The comments I have recorded both during the sessions and under comments, I would voice in the session, interspersed with personal illustrations. Students seem to appreciate my personal sharing. I need to be Liesl wearing the tutor-hat.

Application

The house-drawing exercise: Couples, families, groups, teams.

The gift-sharing exercise: Any closing session.

Comments for whole of Spring Term

We have focused on creativity, on imaging, on art therapy exercises. We have brought person-centred facilitating skills to the images. This is person-centred art therapy.

I have heard it said that all art therapists are person-centred; I have heard the view that by allowing the client the freedom to paint what she wants, you are being person-centred. That is rather a limited definition! My experience tells me that the person-centred way is not modelled to us in our culture, does not come naturally to any of us—however willing we might be to offer it. Much education is required, both in the art therapy world and outside it, to clarify the meaning and implication of the person-centred approach.

May this book help in that process.

I am reminded of my own progression; how, when first introduced to the person-centred philosophy, I understood it, agreed with it intellectually, wanted to operate it at once. And discovered the gap between head and gut: the head understood, the gut had been conditioned by much directive imput, which I was perpetuating automatically: needing to know best, show how clever/helpful I was, solve the problem for others, gain a pat on the head from my invisible mother etc. Much personal work was needed to uproot these old patterns, to become truly available to the person-centred approach in an integrated way. I know that such work is needed in training, before a person can claim to be person-centred. I hope the students have shown such evidence. This, one main purpose of the book. Another, to show the power of images. This, too, I think is being shown. And how the marriage of the two has significant relevance in a very wide setting—not merely in human development, but in a wide area of teaching and training, enabling the person to reactivate her right-side non-verbal intelligence, to know more comprehensively, become more whole.

So often, students report how much they enjoy this term; how each week with each new art therapy exercise, they can make new discoveries about themselves, both as 'client' and as 'counsellor'. Yet I seem to lose this sense of excitement as I record the diverse exercises. I have to settle for the limitation of words—*and* know that the written record is valid: a manual for others.

I note that the group dynamic—not the main agenda—cannot be ignored, is a vital, exciting inevitable component, particularly in this group, with its losses and its ensuing opportunities.

The term consists of several art therapy exercises so that students can experience them for themselves, so that they can practice facilitating, learn from the feedback, relinquish old modes, reinforce new. At the start of the term they found it hard as facilitator, to incorporate the image; they focus on reflecting words, having just grasped the doing of it. Gradually, they hold the mirror up also to the image. They need to make more 'bridges', work more spontaneously, so that the image can give up its message.

Remembering them at the beginning of the year, when listening was hard, I see them, in varying degrees, well on the road of person-centred art therapy. Being with them my own belief becomes yet again reinforced, by the very evidence they bring, that this road is good.

We will see how far we can progress on it next term.

SUMMER TERM
More practice.
Self/peer assessing of portfolios and certificating.

Purpose for whole term

Now the student, as facilitator, can become as creative and spontaneous as the client bringing her image, as, side by side, moment to moment, they embark into the unknown, eliciting the meaning from the image, as a means to more integration, autonomy, and growth. Having learned to swim, she can teach swimming.

Now the student experiences the core of self and peer assessment, as she takes her responsibility in the certificating process.

SESSION TWENTY-FOUR
Watching the whole image making process: Guided Fantasy: Deep Sea Diver

"One lives by mystery and not by explanation."

Purpose

To experience a guided fantasy, to externalise it as a visible image, and to explore it with a person-centred facilitator.

As facilitator, to have the opportunity of watching the entire image-making process and to work with that process, as apt.

To give and receive feedback.

Students acknowledge the long break—they're glad to be back.

I report that Jo is unable to respond to our invitation—yet again—to say goodbye before June 6. We decide that by then we will have moved on too far to reconnect with her leaving, we will be busy with our own process of assessment and ending, we have done our half in asking for a meeting, have taken our half of the responsibility, and we need to leave Jo to take responsibility for her half. We will write to Jo.

We realise, only seven weeks to go!

A reminder about the feedback, which needs to be brought back in two weeks. Each student will write a statement for each student, something like:

'If I came to you for person-centred art therapy, I'd value......and I'd be concerned about......'

These statements will be distributed for inclusion in individual portfolios. The purpose of this feedback is that each student takes responsibility to make a statement about each of her peers. Even if she is not one of her peer's assessors, her comment can be read and taken into account by the assessors. Again, shared responsibility. Students share feelings about preparing their portfolios.

Today is 'part A' of a two week exercise. This week, half the students will be 'counsellor', half 'client'.

The 'clients' will hear a guided fantasy, which they will convey to art form.

The 'counsellors' will have the opportunity, for the first time, to watch the entire image-making process in order to reflect back to the client relevant aspects:

'It took you a long time to begin.'

'You drew this first—this last.'

'You started again—you folded/tore the paper.'

'You went over this several times.'

The *whole* process—not the mere end product—can contain relevant material.

Guided fantasy and art therapy

Several disciplines use guided fantasy: the client follows a fantasy in her imagination, and then talks about it.

I find that by offering the additional component of conveying the fantasy to visible art form, much more material can emerge. The guided fantasy used today is one that I have extended in this way:

Pace of guided fantasy

One common error is to offer a guided fantasy too fast. This can be confusing, even disturbing; you've just about become aware of an image, when you're required to move on. Emotional indigestion can ensue.

I tend to take myself through the guided fantasy which I'm offering, in order to pace myself appropriately. It is better to be too slow than too fast.

Exercise with image 24— Guided fantasy: Deep sea diver
'Close your eyes—relax — and now—you are swimming in a tropical sea, near the shore — you are wearing a diving suit—now you are swimming under the surface, towards the sea bed — looking about you—what do you notice—how do you feel—now you can see the sea bed—as you look about you, you may be drawn to one particular object, plant, creature—whatever — go closer—have a good look — maybe there's something you need to say, or ask this one particular object—maybe it responds—how do you feel —and now it is time for you to be swimming up to the surface again—have a last look round —and now you're swimming up— you've reached the surface— you're swimming back to the nearby shore—you've reached the beach now— You may want to reflect on the swim you've just had—before opening you eyes and coming back to this room. Now convey your fantasy journey in art form, however you need to do this.'

The 'client' students draw, each watched by a 'counsellor'.
Then we divide into two:
Half the counsellors and clients work, watched by the other half of the group in 'observer' position. At the end of the session the observers give the counsellors feedback.
Then we switch over. Those who were observers, now work as counsellors/clients, and the previous counsellors/clients take up observer positions:
Marianne's picture:
Marianne has drawn herself, in black, under the water, swimming towards a seahorse, anemonies, a starfish, some black caves.
I want to chronicle her comments which indicate the emerging issue for her, and for the facilitator.
'At the notion of 'diving' my stomach tightened; I'm afraid of being out of my depth—I'd never contemplate skin-diving,' (yet in the picture she is skin-diving) 'I start to swim under water, I begin to relax—I know I'm safe— there's nothing down there to be afraid of—I panic when I'm afraid—I want freedom from fear.'
Her picture symbolised for her what happens when she goes through fear, relaxes, and discovers there is nothing to

fear. She is under the water. She has an air cylinder—the right equipment for the swim.

It is important to use the symbolic content of the image. In making appropriate 'bridges', the client can relate the picture's symbolic message to her present life. *THAT* is the purpose of art therapy. THEN the picture has disclosed its message. THEN the person can work on the issue.

For Marianne, how to overcome her fear of the unknown, of not being able to breathe; be properly equipped for that which she fears, relax, and discover there is nothing to fear. That she CAN do so—just as she did in the picture. She had a choice—she COULD have stayed on the surface.

The three stages of self-awareness are: knowing, owning, acting.

The picture gives up its gift—so now Marianne *KNOWS* what's around for her that was not in the forefront of her awareness. Now she needs to *OWN* it—work on it with her counsellor, release herself from it, and move to ACTING, to a changed behaviour.

So:

(1) Work with the picture.
(2) Make 'bridges'.
(3) Discover the meaning of the symbolic message.
(4) Work on that issue in the client's life.

Both the person-centred approach and art therapy, invaluable.

Of course, there may have been other themes in Marianne's picture—she is drawn to the starfish.

The starfish says: 'I'm happy just being.' Bridge.

The diver is black—the caves are black—there is a black line between the diver and the underwater life — Bridge.

It helped Marianne to have the whole picture-making sequence reflected to her—which was the microcosm of a well-known strategy of hers to do with fear—fear of the unknown, fear of speaking out—and the need to go through the fear and seeing she's O.K. The image, showing her she CAN do it. *See Fig. 32. (Colour)*

Marianne writes:

Deep Sea Diver

'I placed the diver in last, I'm not sure if it was me but who else could it be.

It would be me if I had more courage. If I had more courage, I would see and enjoy a whole lot more.

The caves were important, the mystery of the unknown, who or what was contained in them? Only if I had courage could I see.

Fear of the unknown but mostly fear of not being able to breathe.

On God, how much of my life have I felt stifled, afraid to speak out, is that what it's all about?' *See Fig. 32. (Colour)*

Comments

Often, as I sit and watch the students produce their unique images, I have a feeling of awe, present as the images are made visible, are being born—none of us knowing what is coming, what is about to be disclosed. To such creations we need to offer much delicate respect, we, the midwives, helping the image from darkness to light, from the unconscious to the conscious. As I watch sometimes I experience something akin to the spiritual.

Application

Widely — in therapy, on training courses.

The purpose of this, as of other guiding fantasy exercises; a vehicle by which symbolic meaning can emerge from the whole symbolic sequence as well as from its individual parts. Facilitators can devise their own exercises as appropriate to their purpose.

SESSION TWENTY-FIVE
Guided fantasy:
Wise old person

"Every creative act involves...a new innocence of perception, liberated from the cataract of accepted belief.'

Arthur Koestler, 'The Sleepwalker'

Purpose

So that those who were 'clients' last week can be 'counsellors' this week, and watch the whole image-making process of the 'client'.

For the 'observer' to watch at work the person(s) she is assessing, and to give clear congruent feedback.

To show how the image, expressed in art form, can take you further than the mere verbal relating of a guided fantasy.

To bring a guided fantasy which can have the potential of a symbolic psychological process—through darkness to enlightenment.

Rosemary brings a query from last week: when she was 'counsellor' making 'bridges', her 'client' did not connect to them, saw no link.

Rosemary thought: 'Shall I use gestalt to get her to see the link?' She chose not to.

Her question: What to do when the client does not make connections for herself?

Answer: Don't push the river.

The counsellor's job is to hold up the mirror. If the client is not ready to look, to see what's in the mirror, accept this, and move on. The counsellor may want to reflect the process if it reoccurs.

'I notice, whenever I make a bridge about tears, you do not connect with it.'

The counsellor needs to ask herself—often!—What is my intention, my purpose? If it is to push the client on so that the *counsellor* feels she's getting somewhere, (as with Rosemary's speculation to use gestalt), desist.

If it is to stay with the client, at *her* pace, you're (both!) O.K.

Exercise with image 25— Guided Fantasy—Wise old person

'—and now, you are in a meadow—looking about you—as you look across the meadow, you see a wood—you are walking towards the wood—you've reached the edge of the wood, and you see a path going into the wood—and now you're walking along this path, into the wood, looking around you—noticing what you see—and how you feel—and now, ahead of you, along the path, you see a clearing, and a cottage in that clearing—you are walking towards the clearing—now you are in the clearing, outside the cottage—you open the door—and go in—as you look about you, you notice a wise old person, welcoming you, seemingly expecting you—and the wise old person says: 'Is there something you want to ask me?'—and you are reflecting on a question to ask——you ask your question—and listen out for a response——how do you feel—now the wise old person says: 'It is nearly time for you to be going, but before you do, I want to give you this gift,'——and you receive your gift, taking a good look at it, noticing your feelings—and now it is time for you to say goodbye, one to the other—and you leave the wise old person and the cottage—and you are back, on the path through the wood—walking towards the meadow—looking about you—what do you see now—how do you feel—and now you're back in the meadow—you may want to find a way of keeping your gift safe so that it is ever available to you—before you open your eyes—come back to this room—and express in artform, your fantasy journey, in whatever way is right for you—

Allow 10-20 minutes (depending on time structure).

This fantasy journey can be a symbolic personal journey, through the dark wood, to the wise person (the wise person within yourself) to gain an answer—both in the answer and the gift — and return, through the wood, often feeling differently—lighter—than on the way in.

It shows that we have within us the capacity to be wise, to know, whenever we want to connect with that aspect of ourselves, to solve a problem, find the way forward. A very power-full, autonomous person-centre process: I DO know for me.

The facilitator needs to be aware of the nature of the journey—leading up to the encounter, the question, the answer, and the gift. Although awarenesses may be gained from any component of the journey, that is its kernel. She needs to know when and where it is appropriate to offer such a theme. It is significant to note, in the picture, whether the person reaches the cottage, asks a question, gets an answer; where she puts herself on the journey—or not. Where is she with her wise self.

Rosemary shares her picture, Kim as her counsellor.

Rosemary: I see the wood close by but have no boundaries between meadow and trees.

Kim: No boundaries between meadow and trees?

Rosemary: Yes—a merging of outer and inner.

Kim: Merging?

Rosemary: Yes, of me and the world around me. My cottage is brown with a thatched roof, but I drew it blue and a shingled roof.

Kim: So there was a change between the inner eye image of the cottage and the drawing of the cottage.

Rosemary: Yes, to make it more magical, something different, unusual; I can make it how I want it.

Kim: Magical is to make it how you want it.

Rosemary: Yes, like with the tarot cards—I want to use the magic in me. My power.

Kim: You've not drawn trees above the roof.

Rosemary: I don't want to fill my space. I need space for me. I saw the hermit inside the cottage but drew him outside.

Kim: So, again, you saw him inside, but changed him, drew him outside.

Rosemary: Yes, I needed to see him better.

Kim: Do you?

Rosemary: Yes, then I could recognise him. He and I are old friends. He is my teacher of inner wisdom.

Kim: So, when you put him where you can see him, you can recognise your teacher in inner wisdom.

Rosemary: Yes, I need to bring the learning about my inner wisdom into the light.

Kim: So you know what's best for you, what you need to do.

Rosemary: Yes.

Kim: You drew the outlines of the hermit faintly and then went over it more boldly.

Rosemary: Yes, I form a faint sketchy outline about anything new, and am firmer when my trust is stronger.

Kim: Is your trust stronger in the hermit?

Rosemary: That's what I want.

Kim: You didn't put yourself in the picture.

Rosemary: Yes, but the hermit is me.

Kim: You and the hermit are the same?

Rosemary: YES! The question I ask is: 'What is outside our universe?' I don't know the answer. To my surprise the answer comes back immediately: 'The same as inside.'

Kim: The same as inside?

Rosemary: Yes—more of the same. Back to my inner wisdom! He presents me with a golden orb studded with jewels.

Kim: Golden orb?

Rosemary: It is a representation of the outer and inner universe. Again, outer/inner. As I carry the precious gift away, the only way I can protect it is to make it invisible.

Kim: Make it invisible?

Rosemary: I usually keep my abilities and beliefs carefully hidden, for fear of ridicule or belittlement—as I have experienced in the past.

Kim: So you hide your precious gift for fear or ridicule

Rosemary: Wow! All I need for a fulfilled life is here inside me—ability, knowledge and belief. There is no need to keep seeking it externally. This is the meaning of all this inner and outer. The answer was within me all along. *See Fig. 33 (Colour)*

The reflecting of the recurring theme of 'inner/outer', the transforming aspects of 'magical', of the process of drawing the hermit, of the missing self, the hidden gift, of her words, all lead Rosemary to the message: to trust the wisdom within herself.

She comments: What a lovely revelation this is for me!

Had Rosemary merely reported her fantasy verbally, much potential material might have been lost. By making the fantasy visible and reflecting back both the process of the image-making and aspects of the image, Rosemary was able to find her 'revelation'.

Kim has made much progress since the beginning of the course. Then, she needed to analyse, get it right; she worried about getting it wrong. Now she is more available to the client, spontaneously reflecting back her world, be this by way of words, image, body, wider reflection, and that which is missing. She trusts herself to put herself aside, be for the client.

Rosemary comments from last week: When counselling Mary, did I use gestalt for my own need to get results, or for Mary. If I'm thinking 'what shall I do here?', it's likely to be for my need; if I offer an intervention spontaneously, in response to my full attention to the client, then it's for the client's benefit. I must be aware of this experiential lesson learned, take it back to work. Self-discovered learning the essence of person-centred counselling!

Comments

This is 'part B' to last week: now all the students—as counsellor—have seen the benefit of working with the whole picture-making process.

As I offer an exercise—particularly one of such powerful potential as today—I am aware of the trust the students place in me, as they open themselves up to their image world: I know the exercise I'm about to offer—they don't. I need to monitor myself, lest I want to gain a false sense of power—or rather, control—from this position.

Application

For anyone needing to re-connect to her wise self, need to resolve an issue, bring unconscious wisdom to awareness.

SESSION TWENTY-SIX
First portfolio exchange
Exercise with Image: Symbol in the round

"It is as if the drawing says for the artist, 'here I am.'
 Nathan Goldstein, *The Art of Response to Drawing*

Purpose

(1) To clarify the certificating procedure. To exchange the first portfolio.

(2) To experience an art therapy exercise where everyone adds to someone's picture. To note what I gave others, what I received, how I felt, and what this tells me about me.

The students have brought in their completed portfolios. I invite comments on how it was to produce them.

Rosemary expresses relief that it's done.

Dawn says it made her keep an eye on herself when working with a client. The discipline helped her to stay with what was going on for her—an important year in her life regarding her own self-awareness.

Kim feels she's been through a lot—it was the most painful experience of her life, keeping a journal. She'll never be the same again, having faced the dark side. An enriching experience.

Heather: For her, it was the first time in her life that she took a look at herself. A most rewarding experience.

Wendy appreciated the discipline of writing the portfolio. It took a long time, she learned and discovered much, and is very satisfied.

Rosemary said it was too precious to show to her family, though she can share herself safely here. So she makes the portfolio 'invisible', like the wise person's gift of last week's exercise.

Others echo this feeling—that the portfolio is too private, too special, to share with near ones outside the group.

I suggest it is important to pause and acknowledge the very real achievement in producing the portfolio; to be pleased with ourselves for the accomplishment, to celebrate. Before attending to the assessment—a pause to value oneself—a model to take to our filofax lives—time to stop, appreciate the self, before moving on to another task.

I comment on the assessment procedure:

(1) That the portfolio being assessed is treated with utmost confidentiality—which means *no-one* away from the group may see it.

(2) The student reads the portfolio, taking account of the group—and the personal contracts, to see if the assessee has, overall, fulfilled the criteria well enough or not. She will make notes as she goes along, and write her assessment at the end. She is assessing the person in the light of the criteria we have set ourselves for the purpose of the certificate, as she knows her from the course, and from her portfolio. She is not taking into consideration personal likes or dislikes of the person—she needs to separate out such feelings. It is the ultimate course experience of being congruent: if the assessor feels that a 'no' is warranted, yet gives a 'yes', she devalues her own and her peer's certificates, and the whole certificating procedure, and denies her assessee important information and a valuable opportunity for learning. Again, the paradox that a 'no' might be the very thing the student needs to hear to move her on.

We note that we are embarking on the ultimate experience of self and peer assessment, leading to—or not—a certificate.

We look at the structure, to be clear as to who takes whose portfolio today.

The assessor's comments are not included in the portfolio yet lest they influence the other assessors. All assessors' comments are included on the assessment day.

We distribute the feedback each student has written for

each student, on the lines of: 'If I came to you for person-centred art therapy, I would value...and I'd be anxious about...'

These are added to the portfolio now.

Such 'friendly information' is of great value: given non-critically, the recipient can allow it in, reflect on it, learn from it.

Exercise with image 26— Symbol in the round
With the time remaining, we decide on a group exercise, to feel connected, together, on this day of portfolio presentation.
Each person takes a piece of paper and puts her name in a corner. We sit in a circle.
Each person draws a simple shape or symbol on her page, then passes it on to her left. Now she adds something to the picture in front of her before passing it on. And so on, all the way round, till her own picture arrives back with her.

(1) Each student comments on her reaction on seeing her picture—with all the additions,

Rosemary: 'I sent out an empty space and I'm annoyed that it got filled up by others.'

Bridge: 'Is that what you do?'

R: 'Yes! When all I want to do really is do things my way, NOT send out an empty space, for others to fill.'

Kim: 'I'm surprised at what's come back to me. It's not in keeping with how I feel.'

'How do you feel?'

'Sad, upset.'

'What did you send out?'

'A bright star.'

Bridge: 'So you feel sad and upset, send out a bright star, and people respond to the bright star; is that what you do?'

'Yes. When I'm not feeling O.K. I'm not congruent with others and then I'm surprised that others can't see I'm not feeling O.K.'

Wendy: 'I don't like these colours—they jar with the rest. There's discord. They spoil the whole picture.'

Bridge: 'So if something jars, if there's discord in a part of your life, it spoils the whole?'

'Yes.'

Mary: 'I'm pleased—all is harmony.'

'So you focus on the harmonious?'

M: 'Well, that's what there is.'

(Her own pictures show mainly the positive not the negative. She is unable to focus on the negative when it is reflected.)

Liesl (who participated today): 'How lovely! I need only do a bit, let others do the rest! I'm not very good at asking for help. This is the wish!' (*This book is about me not doing it all; others contribute!*)

Dawn: 'What a beautiful flower! But this line in the middle spoils it.'

Yes—(*she owns the 'bridge'*)—something central bothering her.

(2) Look around and reflect on your contributions to the pictures of others: what does it tell you about you?

Wendy: 'I complete—make it O.K. for others.'

Kim: 'I put out my anger onto others, whilst not able to express it congruently.'

Marianne: 'I didn't think—I was just spontaneous, did what I want. How I'd like to be!'

Heather: 'I look at the name and give what I think that person wants.' (*A familiar theme*)

And so, yet again: wherever we grab it, however we make images, spontaneously, without thinking, something will emerge about us, how we are, just now, that needs acknowledging.

Portfolios are exchanged.

Symbolically, the tutor has nothing to do with this procedure, which is student-centred.

The tutor gives her feedback, imput, teaching,

throughout the year; now she sits back. The certificating procedure is up to the students.

A key experience of student-centred sharing of responsibility.

We model a radical shift in certificating procedure within the education system. We have our foot in the door!

Comments:

We reach the central aspect of self and peer assessment whereby students take responsibility for awarding (or not) themselves and their peers the certificate. More evidence that when people are given responsibility they behave responsibly.

How do I feel about being redundant at this stage—the course's jewel in the crown—sitting back, not taking any part in the self/peer assessment. A decade ago, probably, I'd have needed to see, know, comment—check if they're doing it 'right'. Now—I'm glad to note—this need has gone. As I step back, others have the chance to know. It needn't be me. Quite a relief! I do have a curiosity to see the portfolios, just to *see* how each student has produced her evidence. I'll be able to take a glance after their certificating procedure.

There are models based on self peer and staff assessment. I prefer, for maximum impact of the experience, to keep out: a tutor's view is given different weight. I prefer to give my views throughout the year, as I teach. Only in my sitting back can the students discover what they do with their power.

Again, an opportunity to see how such a model might be adapted and introduced elsewhere.

I have worked with children who wrote their own reports very honestly, accurately, responsibly. They *do* know about themselves. A teacher writing a report gives the message: I know best about you, reinforcing low self-esteem, as he repeats a familiar message from other settings. We might do well to move towards a system where both teacher and pupil have a say.

I recall a visit to a state school in Holland, where all staff were qualified counsellors, where the ethos of the school was child-centred; pupils involved with decision-making about personal learning issues and the general running of the school: attendance, exam results and ensuing job satisfaction were far above the national average.

QED

Application

Assessment: On any learning programme.

Symbol in round: in any group work, to highlight personal and interpersonal issues.

SESSION TWENTY-SEVEN
Group Mandala

"Symbols are natural attempts to reconcile and reunite opposites within the psyche."

Jung

Purpose

1) For students to experience painting a mandala together.
2) To look at the personal issues which emerge.
3) To look at the group dynamic reflected in the picture.
4) To compare the personal and group position since the time of the group island.
5) To exchange portfolios—the second reading.

Mandala is the Sanskrit word for 'circle'—it is a symbolical diagram, a pattern of existence depicting the dualistic and complementary principles of the universe.

In modern times, Jung re-introduced the use of mandalas as a dialogue between the conscious and unconscious, for use in the field of therapy, stressing the ancient archtypal nature of such drawings.

Mandalas are about balance, wholeness and integration, and can be self-healing as well as self-revealing.

The symbol of the circle denotes unity;

"an expression of the self, and the path to the centre, to individuation."

(Jung: Man and his symbols, p.196)

In drawing a mandala, based on meditation and visualisation, a microcosm of the self will emerge—a photo of the self in the here and now.

Mandalas can be used for groups, to disclose both the dynamic of the individual and of the group.

Today's exercise is to paint such a group mandala, and to see what we can learn from the process.

Exercise with image 27: Group Mandala
We make a large paper circle and put in on the floor. Paints have been put out in addition to the usual crayons, chalks, coloured markers.

The students decide how to use the space: divide in sections? a section for individual and communal work? What? They decide to flow freely anywhere on the circle. There will be half an hour for painting. There are eight students.

Seven students go to fetch paint. Kim stays—starts drawing with chalks.

Mary reaches out from her space to make a mark above Kim's image. She adds to the shapes of all the students—does nothing in the space in front of her, which gets filled by others.

Nina, opposite Mary, stays put in her space.

Marianne puts a yellow circle in the centre.

Kim draws half-way round the circle, then stops.

Rosemary starts last, stops last.

We debrief on an individual level first. Secondly, we will look at the implications for the group.

Kim:

'I had a wonderful time; I wanted to paint, but I wanted to get going, so I used chalk.'

'Does that speak to you?'

'Yes, I want to get going—in my art, for example—I'll follow my energy, rather than delay.'

'You went over the first colour'

'Yes, I wanted it to be bright and happy—to brighten things up.'

'Bright and happy?'

'Yes, usually I use black—I've been in the dark side, and I've come out of it.'

'I got carried away by the process.'

'Carried away?'

'Yes, when I immerse myself—when I paint—I don't think, judge—I just go. I went this far and finished with a snake's head'.

'Snake's head?'

'Yes—not like mother. I know where I am with this snake. It's a nice one, for health.'

Nina:

'I enjoyed using paint. I think the whole has come out beautifully. I felt I could go where I please. I felt safe and had the choice.'

'And you chose to stay in your territory.'

'Yes—but I could choose.'

'Choose?'

'I have a choice now, whatever I do with it. I had bright colours, separately, and I let them merge. I experimented.'

'Experimented?'

'Yes, it's OK to experiment without getting anxious.'

'Anxious?'

'I used to be anxious about trying something new. Less so now.'

'You have not filled in your shapes.'

'No.'

Marianne:

'My first mark was the yellow sun in the middle. I wanted to put in the central core. I would have made it bigger but somebody had made a pattern—so I compromise.'

'Does this procedure speak to you?'

'I don't like being the centre of attention but I want to get in there. I do it my way. And sometimes I need to compromise. I put eight rays. Eight people. I try to keep everybody together. Then I filled in the bits and added.'

'Filled in.'

'I like to see things finished.'

Wendy:
>'I was disappointed—the first colour didn't come out as I'd like it to—not strong enough.'
>
>'Does that speak to you?'
>
>'Yes, I don't express my feelings enough. I could have done with more space.'

Everyone comes in—this is Wendy's theme of the year—more space!
>'Then I connected up.'
>
>'Connected up?'
>
>'Yes, I bring people together. I wanted bright beautiful colours, not dark and muddy.'
>
>'Not muddy?'
>
>'Yes, I get muddy and confused rather than bright and clear.'

Mary:
>'I went to Kim's area and put in an eye with rays from the eye.'
>
>'You had to reach out to get to Kim's space and then you continued, adding to other already given images. You made no marks in your space.'
>
>'Yes, to get out of my deep mood, to balance it, I link with others, away from me.'
>
>'To get out of deep mood, and you put black—the only black used—on the eye in Kim's space.'
>
>'I need to know I'm alive, get away from feelings about death. Put black out elsewhere. My moods change. Again, I'm premenstrual, vulnerable.'
>
>'You've often mentioned your menstrual cycle, and death of your parents.'
>
>'Yes—my moods fluctuate with it.'
>
>'So, one strategy away from your dark mood (your vulnerability) is to be busy with others, put your "black" elsewhere.'
>
>'Yes.'

Rosemary:

'I started last, with white, avoiding dark. Pale is more interesting, subtle, I tell myself. Then I got stronger as I went along.'

'Can you relate to that?'

'Yes, I feel safe, tentative, as I start, and I get more confident as I go along..'

'Then I dared to intrude on Nina's space—(*several reflected Rosemary's issue about her rights to 'intrude' throughout the year—*)

'—then I put the green ring and blue dot in the middle—then I flick paint—then I feel: to hell with it. I go mad! I wanted to spoil it all but stopped myself.'

'What about that whole process?'

'Yes, that's me all the time—tentative at first and then I go overboard at the end—what the hell! And I have to stop myself from going too far.'

'And in this group'

'Hm.'

Dawn:

'I'm annoyed with myself—I wanted to go right in the middle, but Marianne was already there. I wanted to put an imprint of my lips right in the middle, and one for everybody, but I thought you'd think me mad, and I stopped myself. I don't go with my feelings. I censor myself. I wanted to give everybody a kiss, and thought, better not. I withhold love for fear of rejection. I hold myself in, control myself, don't take the risk. That's me. So I do for others (*her old script*) rather than doing what I want.'

'And we're all the poorer for it. We didn't get your kiss, you didn't give it.'

Heather:

'I drew this yellow curving shape—balancing and unfolding.'

'Balancing and unfolding?'

'Yes, that's where I am. Then I needed freedom to move around.'

'Do you?'

'Oh yes! I chose yellow and pink—opposites in a way. Together they made orange. The third position.'

'Third position?'
'Yes, it's not either/or, there's a third position always for me. (*She tends to go from one end of the continuum to the other.*)
'And the eye here'
'Sees and reflects.'
'And your eye?'
'Yes, that's right.

We see again, when talking spontaneously about a drawing, a truth about ourselves will emerge, often revealing an aspect not uppermost in our minds, whatever the art exercise.

Now we review to see what the picture tells us of the group; the role of the individual in the life of the group:

Kim uses chalk—all others paint:
She brings a strong individuality, speaks her mind, can be different.

She started first.

She sits opposite Rosemary, who started last.

Nina is the one in the group who has been self-contained—keeping her feelings to herself—has not filled in her shapes, stayed put.

She sits opposite Mary, who has gone to everyone in the group, has put nothing in the space before her.

Marianne goes to the middle. The one who has quiet courage and confronts for the group. (As at the ratifying session: gentle strength). Her eight rays; she is concerned for all, takes group responsibility.

Dawn wants to go to the centre, show affection, but is ambivalent.

Wendy shows anxiety about setting herself free. She sits opposite Heather, who is gaining her freedom to move around.

Rosemary modelled her pattern throughout the course, starts slowly, gains confidence and is away.

And what about the four who left the group?: No space

for them. We've gone through the pain and grief and rage of loss. We have closed ranks; moved on. Wendy has done a figure of eight; Marianne has eight rays from her sun: now we are eight students. And the tutor? She prepared the circle, gave the circle to the students, upon which to manifest themselves.

It all fits! We are amazed. Yet again that awe-inspiring feeling, as insights surface from the picture, as if by magic. Art therapy.

Wendy has a query: she would have liked to get everyone to start together. This would interfere with the organic process: what each student does, is significant. Rosemary started last, for example, finished last—very much part of her pattern of getting going slowly, then not wanting to stop.

The person-centred way allows the process, in order to gain the maximum learning from it.

As in an individual mandala, here too the balance of opposites emerges. Kim, who starts, opposite Rosemary, who is slow to come in at first, and finishes last. Nina, who keeps to herself, opposite Mary, who goes to everyone. How people sat, therefore, not chance! Amazing. We see the balance of opposites, a central feature of mandalas.

The mandala is useful also to compare: how were we at the time of the group island, how are we now? Four months ago, when drawing the group island, students were responding to Geraldine's leaving, were in touch with their own strategies to loss. This showed clearly on the picture—separate contributions, the need for individual space. Now, on the mandala, the students have worked through four losses, are close, integrated, able to be themselves and with others. All this clearly visible, undisputable. This is us now.

Two group photographs telling their story. The photograph of this group's mandala is on the cover of the book.

The application of such a group exercise is scopeful indeed: families, teams, management. So much can be revealed, so accurately, safely and fast.

The students take home the second portfolio.

Marianne writes:

Mandala

'It was very important for me to be in the centre of it, the light in the centre, yet if you asked me if I like to be the centre of attention. I would say no.

This highlights the dichotomy between aware and unaware.'

Marianne brings this comment about last week's feedback from the group for her portfolio:

'When I received the feedback I felt totally deflated and depressed. The same old messages kept coming through. "Holds back", "lacks confidence". I thought I had improved since last term and, in fact, these comments did not tie in with my self assessment at all. I could not focus on all the wonderful positive things people had written. My response could partly be attributed to pre-menstrual sensitivity. At the same time I *know* I have gained confidence in my counselling skills.'

Heather writes:

Comparison between group island & mandala

'During the island image I was still recovering from Geraldine's departure and felt unable to commit myself completely. I remember making a raft, needing space, feeling overwhelmed by Mary's tree and then tentatively adding things to the island—particularly an underground cave—exploring the unknowns in the group?!

The mandala was a wonderful experience. We seemed to work as individuals but also had a group identity that moved thro' us. I felt I was doing a lot of balancing and supporting patterns and I remember adding the 'crown of thorns' as a symbol of 'the paradox' the imbalance in things that also need to be recognised and the spiritual. It was an amazing experience, a bit like a dance. As I write I am again touched by it all.'

Comments

I feel especially excited watching the emergence of a group picture, because of the unaware inter-personal component that students express in the process of the picture-making. Something magical about watching the unconscious right side intelligence at work before my eyes.

Frequently, archetypal symbols emerge, and whilst the symbol can contain individual meaning, it can also carry some aspect of the collective unconscious.

Today, Kim's snake: she owns the personal level: a snake for health.

What aspects are relevant here of the archtypal: goddesses were ever accompanied by the serpent, depicting the feminine characteristics of intuition; living underground, the serpent is in touch with the dark side. It can be solar and lunar, light and dark, healing and poison, preserver and destroyer. On today's mandala the serpent carried all such archetypal material both for Kim and the group.

The mandala serves two important basic aspects: to restore something from the past and to express something new that does not yet exist. Today we illustrated both these aspects—how an image makes conscious material from the past, and—as I shall show during the assessment session—how a person can already know before the event. In fact, not only mandalas, but all images contain the potential of these two aspects and, like the mandala, the possibility for balance and integration.

Both group and individual mandalas can reveal opposite aspects. So it is with any image: it tends to be a symbolic illustration of some opposite aspect which needs to make itself known. In her aware life a woman is busy being mother, wife, counsellor. Her images repeatedly bring up issues about her autonomy, her identity as a person in her own right. She needs to attend to this message, a balance of opposites making up the whole.

Application

For any group—team, class, family, management—wanting to be aware of its dynamic in order to relate better as well as for individual self-awareness.

SESSION TWENTY-EIGHT
Third portfolio exchange.
Counselling with art therapy 'on the hoof'

"To become an I, I need a thou.'

Martin Buber

Purpose

An opportunity to offer art therapy spontaneously within a counselling session.

The students prepare the rota for next week's assessment session: 20 minutes per group, 40 minutes to de-brief. Today they take home the last of the three portfolios.

A reminder about the procedure:

The assessment will determine—based on the student's portfolio and the student's presence in the group—whether, overall, she has or has not met the three main criteria:

Showing personal development;

showing understanding of the theory both of the person-centred approach, and of art therapy;

showing the ability to use person-centred art therapy skills both on the course and in a work setting.

The certificate is based on on-going self and peer assessment: this, the final assessment, the ultimate opportunity to take responsibility, to be congruent, to say both the positive and the negative—a key part of the year's experience.

Exercise with image 27: Introducing art therapy 'on the hoof' within a counselling session
So far we have experienced specific art therapy exercises, to see what can emerge from the image for ourselves, and to practice facilitating skills.
Today the structure is more spontaneous: the client talks to the counsellor. When the counsellor intuitively knows that the opportunity is there, she sug-

gests imaging and drawing that image. She works with the image, moves on to verbal counselling as appropriate.

Imaging can be particularly helpful with *feelings*.

'Close your eyes—see if an image comes to you of your anger.'—The image itself, and the drawing of it, can put the client more immediately in touch with that feeling than mere 'talking about'—which is once removed, cerebral reporting.

With *symptoms;* to allow an image of the pain, the cancer, the fracture—again the actual image, the portraying of it, the talking about it spontaneously, can help the client to experience and express feelings about the symptom with more immediacy, and paradoxically, lead to healing.

With *addictions*, with *victims of abuse;* imaging can be a powerful way to confront the unspeakable.

A particular *situation* can evoke important images, possibly connect to earlier times, patterns.

'See what image/memory comes to you about this scene.'

With *emotive words*: 'you say you feel abandoned; close your eyes; what image comes to you as I say 'abandoned'?' Working in this way, the counsellor can be at her most spontaneous and creative. The more she sets aside thoughts (should I come in now) the more she trusts her intuition in the moment, the more likely she is to work resourcefully with her client.

This mode of working is of particular relevance in one-to-one counselling.

So far the students have seen how quickly an image gives up its message. Combined with counselling, there is the opportunity to work on that message.

The students decide to work in pairs, for half an hour each way, with 10 minutes for feedback, followed by sharing in the group.

Marianne describes a situation at work. Two colleagues are in conflict. each in turn comes to her to talk to her about the problem, as does the boss. One bit of Marianne wants to listen in a person-centred way, allow the individual to explore and work through the problem.

Another bit of her feels she has to solve the problem for them, find a solution. 'See if an image comes up for your about these two parts of you.'

She draws a brick wall, with yellow light behind the wall, and an orange circle in the centre.

The brick wall stops her light from shining fully—the light of wisdom and insight. The orange circle is warmth.

The wall is about the fear of being invisible. It leads Marianne on to recall how, as a child, she felt invisible, unheard, when she wanted attention from her parents about a problem and didn't get it. 'If only they'd tell me what to do.' So, her formula of being visible became telling someone what to do.

In order to be visible, needed, she becomes the rescuer, problem-solver, keeping others in 'victim' position. And she doesn't want to do it: 'You're an adult—work it out yourself,' crossly. From 'persecutor' corner. She knows she needs to get out of that old triangle—rescuer, persecutor, victim—even if it's risky, may alter relationships.

Afterwards, Marianne reports that she had no idea that her image was connected to the problem—not till she talked about it. The more you allow a spontaneous image to emerge, the less you illustrate a 'thought', the more likelihood of discoveries.

During feedback on the exercise:

Wendy—says it helped her to focus on the feeling, express it.

Heather—says it helped her be more specific. It was important to experience it for herself, now she can offer it to others.

Nina—says it was more intense, weaving words and picture, reaching a deeper level.

Rosemary—reports on the luxury of being heard.

Dawn—owns that, as the counsellor, she did not stay where the client was (issue about a person at work), made her own assumptions and got her to image about boundaries—an issue of her own. A mis-match ensued, preventing Rosemary from focusing on *her* problem.

Reflect—that's enough! Your own speculations intrude, are not person-centred.

To make up numbers, I participated:

I was left feeling: if only I had someone to hear me for half an hour each day, how well I would be! Today's half hour uncovered, via a symptom, bits of my process to which I was not paying attention.

We are too busy with content, don't allow on-going time for process. At our peril.

In the time remaining we acknowledged the imminent ending of the course. What are our strategies re endings, loss or change? Are they appropriate now?

Wendy: It's not an ending—a beginning. I'll do something else—needn't travel—I've gained a lot here.

She acknowledges the positive, not the negative. Owns that this might be her strategy. Denial of the ending.

Marianne, too, says she tends to deny the sadness of endings.

Heather knows she'll suffer, it'll be painful.

My own strategy was to withdraw before the ending—get in first to avoid rejection. Memory of endings of long ago—and the ensuing pain—would motivate my behaviour. Having worked on the original trauma, I am more able now to be in the present.

When there is enough time, this theme lends itself well to imaging: 'Close your eyes—what picture comes up for you around—endings—loss—change.' A deeper level of awareness may be reached.

Rosemary brings this about her role as assessor.

'I had no anxieties about assessing until I received a portfolio that presented me with a problem. I had not envisaged that I may have to tell someone that they were not in my opinion eligible for the Certificate. I struggled with this dilemma for two weeks trying to avoid making a final decision, trying to find a way round a difficult situation, trying to ignore the discomfort that my conclusion brought with it. I wanted to discuss it with someone, let them decide for me; in short I wanted to avoid the burden of this responsibility, to give away my personal power. The power was only OK for the positive task, not for the negative one. I had to force myself to look at this. Eventually I stayed with the discomfort, trying to discover why I was feeling so bad about it. Did I fear a confrontation with the person I had negatively assessed? Or any possible recriminations from other group members? Or was I identifying with a dread of receiving negative feedback myself? Would I expose myself to negative evaluation and judgement from others? Was I being truly congruent in my assessment or was there left over business from the group sessions? I had to explore and answer all these angles before I arrived at the conclusion that my decision must stand. I could not back out or avoid, which would have been so much easier to do, to search for a few positive aspects and ignore all the negative ones. I still find it much more difficult to give negative information than to receive it—I suppose I am far more used to receiving it. I had to re-evaluate my position as an assessor in the light of my learning processes on this course, otherwise then I would not have benefitted from it as much as I kidded myself I had. That was quite a revelation in itself. An excellent test for myself to finish the year. I saw that in order to be fully congruent I must take responsibility for my actions. In practice this is far harder than in theory. I must present the negative feedback fully, honestly and without fear of the possible consequences. It is central to the person-centred model. This has been an uncomfortable, but nonetheless enriching experience that I am sure will benefit me in the long term. Thank you, Carl Rogers.

Comments

This is where we take off the water-wings, and swim freely. No need for a device for imaging.
 I watch, with pleasure. Like a parent who has helped and encouraged the child to walk, seen the first steps, the faltering, the falls, and now, there's the child, striding out, knowing how. Of course there's much walking still to do, without me there; along muddy paths, down slippery slopes, up precarious mountainsides, through glorious country lanes, but the basic walk has been learned. So the term—and my task—can come to an end.
 Talking about, can keep one in the left-side thinking mode. By spontaneously incorporating art therapy with the verbal component, deeper truths may be revealed, and progress towards integration may occur.

Application

For counsellors, therapists, art therapists, expressive art therapists working one-to-one, and in their training.
 For use with addicts, terminally ill, abused, bereaved, cancer patients, HIV sufferers, etc.
 In fact, for any client where words are inadequate to reach the central issue.

SESSION TWENTY-NINE
Assessment

"Learning is finding out what you already know. Doing is demonstrating that you know it. Teaching is reminding others that they know just as well as you. You are all learners, doers, teachers."

Richard Bach, *Illusions*

Purpose

Each student has read the portfolios of three peers whom she is assessing.

Students meet to give their feedback, based on the student's portfolios and the experience of that student throughout the course. Has the student met the course criteria well enough overall to gain the certificate—or not? They experience perhaps the hardest test of the year, of being responsible and congruent—the kernel of the course. They participate in collective power-sharing, a very different model to the one generally used in education. They flatten the pyramid of authority: the political aspect of the person-centred approach. They can see where else such a model can be applied. How to effect change in other systems. They see the importance of dealing with feelings left after the certificating process.

Mary announced she would be absent for the last session. We would leave 10 minutes at the end for farewells.

Each student is to spend twenty minutes with her assessors, as per the rota drawn up last week, to receive feedback, evaluation and assessment regarding her certificate.

After this there would remain an hour for comments, and for Mary's leave taking.

After the completion of the assessment, each student reported her result.

Mary: 4 'yes'.
Nina: 2 'yes'—2 'no' (i.e. no certificates).

Nina is upset, wants to challenged the decisions. We decide to go round each student first.

Dawn:	4 'yes'.
Wendy:	4 'yes'.
Marianne:	4 'yes'.
Rosemary:	4 'yes'.
Heather:	4 'yes'.
Kim:	4 'yes'.

We return to Nina, agree to divide the time between Nina, and to debrief the remaining assessment experience.

Rosemary—who said 'no'—said that Nina had not fulfilled her personal contract: no evidence of personal development; no theory input.

Wendy—who said 'no'—said Nina had not included the learning of the sessions and there was no evidence of learning of the theory—two of the three main criteria missing.

Kim, the third assessor, had given a 'yes'. Nina had given herself a 'yes'.

Nina felt that her assessors were 'nit picking', She did keep a journal (waved it), but it was just for her—nor had she included her reading list (evidence of theory—or shown understanding of theory). She wanted the journal to be considered now.

Liesl mentioned the taking of personal responsibility in meeting the group contract—what needed to be included, shown.

Also, that the group had made no provision for an appeals procedure. Nina seems to be appealing to have her journal considered now.

On this, a short part-time course, the students have been clear since devising their certificating structure that the certificating procedure in the penultimate week was the final hurdle in their self/peer assessment, and that they needed to take responsibility accordingly.

Nina comes in quickly:

Could Wendy read her journal by Saturday. Wendy agreed. Liesl reflects this exchange.

There is no response from other group members. The tutor reflects this too.

It is 15 minutes before the end. Has there been a quick rescue job, without examining the process? To end well? Deny the learning of the congruent 'no'?

Could this be a familiar strategy?

Next week is the last session.

I remember how the Xmas celebration was hijacked by 'a student'. Will we be denied our ending by Nina? Will we be finished or unfinished? Will the group take responsibility? I hold back, trusting that they will.

We go on to debrief the certificating of the other students. Possibly the first time the students have participated in such an educational process.

How was it?

Heather: It was nerve-racking as the assessor, and good to be understood as the assessee.

Mary: It felt good to be understood. It was a privilege to read other people's personal sharing and difficulties.

Marianne: It was a tremendous responsibility.

Kim: I felt moved and privileged to read about such courage and honesty.

Wendy—appreciated the honesty. She was anxious regarding the responsibility.

Dawn—went through the whole gamut of emotion, to reach the objective position of not allowing the personal to interfere.

She was relieved not to have to say 'no'.

Rosemary—felt the responsibility of saying 'no'.

The tutor symbolised her position during the procedure by sitting alone in the course room (whilst students, in other rooms, assessed one another), acting as time-keeper of the 20 minute slots.

As tutor, to operate this model, to sit back, to allow

others their power, means the ability to relinquish control, the need to have a say. And to feel OK about sitting back, letting others be.

Time is up: we decide to say goodbye to Mary on Saturday. Students leave their portfolios behind, so I might get a glimpse of them by Saturday.

Symbolically, I as tutor see the portfolios after the certificating procedure.

Rosemary writes:

'When Nina wanted to appeal, things were happening much too fast for me to respond properly. I wanted no part in an appeals system. We had all set up the goal posts. When someone missed the goal, the group appeared suddenly willing to move the goal posts to allow that member to score, to provide a fairytale ending. If Nina gets her certificate through the back door, I felt that my certificate and everyone else's would be devalued as a result.'

Heather writes:

'I certainly valued the 'theory' of the p-c approach before your course but I am sure I did not clearly appreciate it as I hadn't experienced it personally. It has been the 'doing of it' myself that has been so important to me, as it has enabled me to 'know' this for myself and therefore trust it. I don't mean this only in the work setting but in terms of a good model for everyday living. Sometimes, particularly, in the beginning I didn't always have enough courage in my own power to speak clearly. I am surprised how this is so much easier for me now. Self-assessment has been easier than peer assessment. It is not so easy to say something negative, but helpful to peers in the group. I have recognised though that the negative things others have been prepared to say help me, so I have got on with it.

Looking at the portfolios has been a privilege as they are often so personal and touching and such records of growth—it is difficult to be critical of this, like criticising someone's baby but that's what we agreed to do. I have tried to get on with it.

Self and peer assessment—I found this a significant part of the person-centred approach in that it was the way in which we had to confront taking responsibility. I remember this started for me on the 'group contract day' when I took a long time to confront 'a student' in stating how I felt about the contract. I grew thro' that and the fact that you (Liesl) didn't intervene and so I had to in the end. Again on the day of personal contracts I was so thrown by 'a student's' personal contract that even tho' I wasn't in her ratifying group I did say to her that if I had to assess her in the end I wouldn't be able to accept it. When you are given responsibility you have to face your own integrity in the end. It is an uncomfortable and tough experience this type of assessment but once committed to it ensures full participation. It is much tougher than 'unfaced authority' assessing one from above.

I came to the course to gain something, I gained more than that—tools to use with others—yes! but more importantly an important nudge inwardly for myself.

Thank you Liesl for your part in all of that.'

Marianne writes:

'For me, assessing other group members' work has been *difficult*, *disturbing* and *rewarding*.

It has been *difficult* because I want to do justice to the peer assessment procedure and this requires much soul searching. How can one be totally honest without hurting someone. How valuable congruent feedback is; I appreciated it and I hope I have been able to give it to others ('a student' did not appreciate my feedback, it caused a barrier between us). It is a tremendous responsibility.

It has been *disturbing* because I keep thinking how much better than mine other people's portfolios are, how much more time they have put into it, how much more precise. I did what I could, what I thought was enough, I had nothing to compare it with—until I saw and read the others. 'Why didn't I do that?' 'Is mine good enough?' If I feel what I have done is good enough, have I demonstrated it adequately?' Old worries impede.

It has been *rewarding* and a privilege to share other group members' work, insights, fears, successes and failures—their view of what has transpired in the group and the variations in the work settings. I have been inspired by the openness and honesty of the participants.'

Kim writes:

'Personal and peer assessment was my greatest single lesson in being congruent. It also ensured that I worked harder than I had ever done on any course (school, college, etc) because there was no examiner or exam to blame at the end. As a group we had defined the contract and the content of the portfolios. We had not set an arbitrary pass mark or a quantifiable goal, i.e. no. of pages, no. of hours, etc. If the criteria were not met well enough then the certificate would not be awarded.

I found myself in the assessment group that, I think, had the hardest time. Two out of the three of us found one portfolio lacking. I had passed it. Although I was aware that the content was thin and some aspects were missing, I knew how dedicated and committed my colleague was and so felt had earned the certificate. I found this episode very hard and still do. So many conflicting feelings came and went during the couple of weeks of assessing this particular portfolio, making it very difficult for me to be congruent with myself and others. I learnt so much from this, our final hurdle.'

After the session, Rosemary rings. She is upset about the rushed 'appeals' procedure—no discussion, no agreement. She sticks to her 'no'., unwilling to change the goal posts.

Wendy rings: despite reading the journal she still feels that Nina has not fulfilled her personal contract; she needs to take responsibility for leaving out the journal—clearly relevant evidence. Also, there is no mention of understanding the theory; still one main area missing. She is saying 'no'. She did her usual 'thing' of agreeing too quickly. There had been no consensus for the 'appeal'. And only she—one of the assessors—to read the journal? That's not on.

(At the receiving end of the 'phone, I reflect and clarify their comments.)

Each will give Nina her repeated 'no' when she rings.

Later, on the Moderator Day, Kim—the third assessor—was able to tell the group that she allowed her wish for Nina to receive the certificate to come before her objective congruent appraisal.

Comments

What a session! Again, the main learning through that which was difficult: the one 'no'.

Even if this course ends, our journeys continue. We have the possibility to take the learning on with us. Often the feedback, regarding a 'no' to the certificate, is what we need to hear. Paradoxically, those who get a 'no' get the potential of the biggest gift. A hurried 'appeals' procedure may rob them of this gift.

On some level Nina sabotaged herself—getting herself rejected before being rejected—by not fulfilling the contract. At the same time she desperately wanted the certificate, pleads for an appeal, criticises her assessors.

I remember Nina's contract, where she writes that she will take responsibility for that which she decides to include. I remember the group mandala, where Nina keeps to herself—within the circles not filled in, and her comment that she had a choice to go—or not to go—where she pleased. She chose to stay in her own space. Self-contained. Not to share. On the course as in the portfolio. Choice equals responsibility. I remember pointing out to her my concern about her incomplete contract during the ratifying session—the very purpose of astringent ratifying, to avoid a situation such as Nina's at the certificating session. I hope, since the course, she might have been able to look at her 'gift', about taking personal responsibility.

Rosemary's process on the mandala—intruding on Nina's space—illustrates an amazing aspect of imaging, that the image, not bound by chronological sequence, can impart information *before* an event. Intuitive knowing. The more we come to accept this knowing, the less amazed we'll be. Rather, we'll say: But of course!

Some people question the tutor role in this model: what if the students get it wrong. This occasion yet again shows very dramatically that the model works: By allowing the process, Wendy and Rosemary, on reflection, could return to the congruent and difficult decision of giving Nina a 'no', despite the temptations to rescue. Each had an opportunity to learn much: Wendy has a tendency to agree too quickly, deny her own power. She was able to reclaim it. Rosemary—as shown on the group mandala—may start slowly, but in the end, spoke out with courage and honesty. In group terms, Rosemary and Wendy fetched us out of the VPR triangle, to a level way of being. Other group members learned much about their silent collusion.

Rosemary and Wendy gave the certificate its worth, for an unwarranted 'yes' would devalue the certificate for each recipient. I have found over and over again, with diverse age groups, in diverse situations, that when one gives the message: 'I trust you, I believe in your capacity to behave responsibly', then people behave trustworthily and responsibly. As here. Even if, now and again, an inappropriate decision is made—no scheme is perfect: in the conventional mode the examining tutor can err also. Overall, the student centred model, based on care-full, thought-full, respect-full congruent feedback of several peers who have known, worked with, and observed the assessee closely for a whole year, and who have a very clear understanding and awareness of the certificating criteria involved, is to be, in my view, preferred.

This certificating model is important politically—relinquishing control, sharing responsibility, in an education setting. Students had a powerful experience of it—much more real and immediate than theorising. Now they can reflect how they can transpose such a model, introduce it to other settings. Initiate change. That is the potential of the course, of the person-centred way.

I'm exhausted! I find being actively engaged in a passive way can take more energy than participating! I'm at the most risk here, to regress; intervene, know best; in my need to be liked, to have a good outcome, I could take control, and deprive others of the opportunity to discover for themselves. I need to be aware of my inner process whilst at the same time tuning in to whatever is happening around me. Overall, I think I held back sufficiently today, whilst the students had the opportunity to make their own discoveries.

This, the struggle, and the reward, of the student-centred tutor, who aims to allow self-discovered learning, aims to empower others.

Application

Any learning situation.

Any group operating shared decision-making, self-peer assessment. student-centred learning.

THE MODERATOR DAY
Dialogue with the Moderator

"Do not follow where the path may lead. Go, instead, where there is no path, and leave a trail.'

Purpose

For the three student groups—of which the 'book' group is one—to come together, as part of one course.

For the Crawley College moderator to meet with the students.

For the students to see the symbolic importance of an education authority incorporating a student-centred mode of certificating.

For an opportunity to welcome visitors.

For celebration of the day, the participants, the work.

Someone has telephoned for Nina, to say she won't be coming today or Wednesday; her baby is ill.

The three student groups come together to meet one another, and Anne Cathcart, the course moderator.

Her task, to be a bridge between Crawley College and the course members; to check out with them, how they devised and carried out their group contract and assessment procedure.

She needs to satisfy herself that this, the student-centred mode of certificating, was carried out responsibly enough to warrant Crawley College certificating the course.

To me, this is an important component of the course: that an education authority shows interest in, and allows, an alternative, radically different mode of certificating; one where the students themselves, rather than those in 'authority' take responsibility to agree on and implement assessment and certificating criteria and procedures. The political aspect of the person-centred way in action.

Anne introduces herself and clarifies her role.

Students go into small groups, preferably with students not from their own course group. They reflect on their contract-making, assessing and certificating procedures, as a way of focusing themselves on the task.

Then, in the large group, Anne questioned each course group about their structure.

The Monday 4-6 pm group was the one to decide on support groups, meeting twice each term, outside course time.

They chose two ratifiers for the personal contract.

Their criteria for assessment were based on 'good enough'.

Students note how, within much similarity, differences emerged.

From the Monday 7-9 pm group

1) Students discovered the responsibility to their peers; they attend, not just for themselves, but also, to be available to assess their peers.

2) The importance of experiential learning. No amount of reading can replace the participating in—say—the contract-making day. Then, only then, you truly know. The value of learning by doing.

The Wednesday group (the group of this book) next:

They used the course brochure, and certain of its 'givens', as a basis for the group contract.

Kim had struggled, having to balance 'anything goes' with limitations, to take responsibility realistically.

Heather reported how long it took her, on the contract-making day, to stand up to the student who exercised much control.

For Marianne, it was an important occasions, when she stood up to 'a student' during the ratifying procedure. Neither she, nor Kim ratified this student's contract, who, then, left the course.

Wendy reported shifting from an 'I'm alright Jack' attitude, to taking responsibility in the group.

The group ratified their personal contracts in two groups of six.

Heather learned the most through the most painful.

Kim guessed that members brought much outside luggage to the group, adding to the fraught dynamic.

Rosemary said she had thought through issues much further than in other settings.

The group decides that it needs more time to 'debrief' Nina's not getting the certificate—in its own session next week.

This is the group that lost most members (four) this year, or any year so far. (As I write, none of this year's 36 students have left.)

Wendy said she found 'negative' criticism, caringly given, most helpful. 'Friendly information.'

Heather felt some of the students, who subsequently left, tipped much blaming onto the tutor. She liked the level way in which the tutor dealt with these—liked the model and learned much from it.

The tutor reported the importance of supervision, particularly at such times.

Dawn spoke of the importance, in assessing, to assess the person vis a vis the contract, rather than the whole person, her likes or dislikes of that person. She said: I had to own all my own imput. I have a sense of achievement like nothing I've every felt before. Learning from books is 'easy'—yet superficial. This was difficult, and I've achieved a great deal.

The Wednesday group acknowledging the paradox that through the losses, the pain, the difficulties, they had the potential to gain the most. This emerges also as we look at the three mandalas (all three on display round the room), and how they inter-relate; what, in terms of the whole course community, each group—unknowingly—carried for the other two. A fascinatingly magical aspect of art therapy.

The 'Wednesday' mandala reflects loss and pain, as well as celebration. Life and death, a balance of opposites. It illustrates the group journey—mirroring the therapy process itself—of going into the dark side before being able to grow. Life, death, and resurrection.

The Wednesday group has definite, rather than abstract shapes: eyes—to see, in and out—yin/yang, several 'eights' to acknowledge: we are eight. Four have gone. OK. And we're OK. The Wednesday group carried the 'no'—the ability to fail someone—for the whole course. This one 'no' in my view earns the course its Crawley certificate. All is paradox! Through pain comes strength and courage. The ability to stand up and be congruent. The Wednesday group used the strongest colour: both the cerebral and the intuitive represented.

Kim was sorry the tutor was not on the mandala.

She gave the paper—the space.

Her task, to be available to the process, to reflect back the whole.

The Monday 4-6 group mandala, with each member separate, had harmony and cooperation also. No-one left in this group—so perhaps, that others could leave.

The Monday 7-9 group mandala showed the balance of the lateral and vertical, and much harmony; both.

It is time for lunch.

Shared lunch in the garden. The generous, carefully prepared dishes brought by each student, a symbolic reflection, how students value the course and one another. Two of our advisory Council guests—Brigid Proctor and Francesca Inskipp, join us and are introduced.

Brigid Proctor, freelance counsellor/trainer and consultant, convenor of the Training Committee, British Association for Counselling. Founder of the first counselling course based on self-managed learning. Brigid was my tutor when I was a student on that course. Later, I too was a tutor there. It is apt that she is here today.

Francesca Inskipp, freelance counsellor, trainer and supervisor, member of BAC training committee and courses recognition group. A pioneer in the world of humanistic psychology, her tape on counselling skills still one of the best of its kind.

Later, Brian Thorne joined us. Director of Student Counselling at the University of East Anglia, and a partner in the Norwich Centre for Personal and Professional Development. He is the co-author of Person-Centred Counselling in Action; one of the banner bearers of the person-centred approach in Britain.

A formidable trio, indeed, to visit us and see our work!

After lunch, Anne, the moderator, sees six students and their portfolios for 20 minutes each.

Meanwhile, half the students talk with our guests, and the other half participate in an art therapy exercise with me—in two one-hour slots, with a changeover after one hour, so that all can do both.

Exercise with image 28: Getting out of a box
Here is the art therapy exercise:
'You are in a box...what is it like there? What's the box made of...what is its size...how do you feel...?
...and now it is time for you to be getting out of the box...what do you do...how do you feel?
...now you are outside the box...look at it now...look around you...how do you feel...? Now look ahead of you, in the direction you might now be going...what do you see...ahead of you...in the distance...?
...when you're ready, draw your experience.

The students decide to work in pairs, or threes, with someone from another student group. For some, the issue was, the ending of the course. For some, their personal journey, or a particular part of it.

Then we all gather for Anne's summary. She is impressed, sees development and growth, diverse and creative work. Certainly, the criteria are met, to satisfy Crawley

College regarding the certificate. She will bear back this message with conviction.

Our guests, too, comment; Francesca is impressed by the amount of work covered in the year, by the potential of images. Brigid likes the integration of both left and right side of the brain. Brian is congratulatory of the course. A good time for our celebration tea—one group baking the cakes, one bringing fruit, and one providing Pimms with which to toast the course. A true and apt celebration to mark the end of the day, and academic (?)—experiential!—year.

I am well satisfied.

A special day.

Anne Cathcart, in her Moderator's Report, was well satisfied that the course criteria had been met. She concludes:

"This is a unique training programme. No other course in Britain can offer students anything like this approach. I believe that it is very important that Crawley College should continue to offer support to this project. The College gains in prestige as a result of its association with it."

Comments

The group felt safe enough to share its difficulties—and successes—with the other groups—and then continued to debrief the process about their certificating—an organic way forward, clearing the way for our ending. I am amazed how much they've learned—and are demonstrating—about congruence. In fact, throughout this year, I've felt, I needn't do anything, the students are bringing the proof. The point of the book.

Kim speculated that students bring much outside luggage to the group: I share this view:

Paradoxically, when students feel safe, they can re-enact old patterns here. Some students are unable to become aware of their projections, some can make the connections, free themselves of old outmoded strategies and incorporate healthier, more relevant ways of being. Often such re-enactments are projected onto me—the aspect of the work I find hardest—separating out that which is mine, that which is not. My own supervision of vital importance to me here. And yet, these very difficulties offer potential for the most learning and growth. As the members of this group discovered again and again during the year. So, in retrospect, I am glad to have chronicled a group which had to weather much storm in order to bask in the sun. Again, the feeling of 'of course—it had to be this group.' Perhaps I knew without knowing.

The day brings together diverse strands of the year: As the moderator questions, the students can review the year's experience.

They have worked in their group. Now they meet the students of the other groups; they see there are more of us.

So far we've been self-contained. Meeting the moderator and our guests enables us to see our work vis a vis others. On this occasion, others who though new to our work, are supportive and encouraging of it. In the real world, innovations may encounter a less encouraging response; we may need to explain, demonstrate, educate. Even then old beliefs, prejudices and fears can get in the way of dialogue. There is excitement, and frustration, for the pioneer.

So, patience: we are making inroads, are being heard and valued more and more, as we share our evidence with enthusiasm and conviction. As today.

As I clear up the house—and garden—I notice yet again that when I'm spending my energy in a position way, I feel less drained, and even my fatigue is tinged with exuberance.

Application

All student-centred models of learning.

SESSION THIRTY
Ending

"A life without celebration is only half lived."

Z. Budapest. *The Grandmother of Time*

Purpose

To deal with any unfinished business.

To take stock: what I've gained from the course, where I am, where I need to go.

To acknowledge the ending of the course—the group—with its feelings.

To celebrate.

To say farewell. Fare well.

I hand out information about the Person-centred Art Therapy Association. This was formed by students five years ago: they wanted an opportunity to have continuing contact, after the end of the course. The Association offers some three workshops per year, with an AGM and a newsletter for exchange of views and information. Several regional groups have formed where members meet for support, sharing, and supervision. An organic outcome of the course.

Kim wants to continue with the post-certificate course.

This course, too, emerged, based on the demand of those students who, at the end of the first year, felt the need to reinforce the learning. As there is no certificate at the end, the year offers the experience of learning for its own sake. This is freedom to learn in the person-centred mode for its own sake, as Rogers, who did not believe in qualifications, had envisaged. Students can develop and increase their skills, bring issues from work, try out new initiatives, explore other media (clay, poetry, music, myth, ritual). The structure is flexible, to meet on-going requirements, the experience rich. As tutor, I enjoy the liberty—without the restrictions and criteria of a certificate—to respond to the need of the now.

For this year's annual report for the course's Advisory Council, I want to collate the students' own comments. I ask for their comments—the students agree. Spontaneously they each write a brief statement:

> 'The PCAT course has helped me to know myself better as a person and also enable me to consolidate and acquire new skills as a counsellor. The best course I have ever been part of.'
>
> Dawn.

> 'This course is about personal growth but you certainly add to your tools professionally along the way.'
>
> Heather.

> 'I have learned more about myself in the last year on the person-centred art therapy course than in the previous 40 years of my life.'
>
> Rosemary.

> 'The art therapy course has enabled me to develop at my own pace in my own way in a non-threatening yet challenging environment.'
>
> Marianne.

> It was a great experience—at times a struggle to keep with it—but so rewarding to have completed it.'
>
> Wendy.

> 'This year changed my life. If I walked down the street today and saw myself at the beginning of the year walking towards me, I wouldn't recognise myself!'
>
> Kim.

Mary is away.

I thank the students for their contributions to the book. I thank them for letting me look at their portfolios: each so creatively unique, bringing evidence in such varied ways.

Such diligent work; eight amazing self portraits. Awe-inspiring.

Now to de-brief the assessment session, and Nina's failure to gain a certificate.

We need to take personal responsibility for the process.

Dawn felt: there but for the Grace of God go I—and therefore colluded with the rescue of Nina.

Heather did a rescue in agreeing to have Nina's journal produced and read.

Wendy agreed to read the journal—a familiar rescue response, without reflecting.

Liesl, in sitting back and trusting the process, got back a huge gift, reinforcing her belief that a system based on Roger's key concept that a person can reach her/his potential when seen as trustworthy, WORKS.

The students have discovered the validity of this concept for themselves in a dramatic way.

Kim, who gave a 'yes', knew the work did not meet the group contract criteria, but rescued herself and Nina by disregarding this knowledge, focusing on the evidence in the case studies.

Marianne, way back at the ratifying process, knew Nina's contract was incomplete, but as she was preoccupied challenging 'a student', she rescued herself—let the contract go through.

Rosemary, congruent, was angry at the 'changing of the goalposts'—talk of appeals procedure without agreement or structure—and subsequent bi-lateral deal between Nina and Wendy, which could have made nonsense of the procedure, and de-valued the certificate.

Much evidence, what happens when one gets caught up in the dreaded triangle—and how two of the group disengaged themselves from it. We reflect on the year's journey. Today, the remaining six bear witness to the paradox that, having worked through so much difficulty, in the end, they learned and gained the most.

We acknowledge that somehow, since last week, when we left with much distress and uncertainty, we worked through the process—largely on the moderator day—to feel strong and clear and sure and OK now. And very close.

We comment on the moderator day: a good experience, using the coffee break to debrief the certificating session, and move on. Good to know of the other groups, a sense of a pioneering network. Good to be validated by the moderator and our guests. A vital part of the whole course. A rich varied day both in content and process.

A celebration.

Exercise with image 29: Stocktaking
Now an exercise, with imaging, and art, to reflect on the course's experience. A stock-taking.
'You are a traveller, on your journey. Last September this journey brought you here, to this course; you came here each week for a year.
Reflect—take yourself back over the year—what did you learn?
Perhaps an image, a symbol comes up for you—what are you taking away with you—what is your harvest—on this Summer Solstice?
And what might you be relinquishing, leaving behind?—let an image come—
Where are you now on your journey—and, though this course is ending, where does your path lead now?
When you're ready, convey this journey on paper.

Marianne:
Draws a dark 'stalk' At the beginning I felt dark—feared the unknown. It was difficult—the stalk gets greener.

Heather: After the difficulties the stalk turns green.

Marianne: Yes, the hard bits lead to growth—and the multi-coloured flower at the top—blowing its seeds into the future. This cloud of self-doubt is in the past. Now there's sun. And here, space for the unknown. I no longer fear it.

Dawn:
This is the tunnel I was in. Dark—moments of light—I feel alone and lost. Having ventured into the light, I have found a whole new side of me—this, the pink, a balance to

the grey. A yin-yang. I've come away from the tunnel, towards the light. With two level, balanced loads, integrated—the new and the old me.

Wendy:

This green line is the journey of ups and downs, highs and lows. I got off the page on a high.

Here I am now, arms extended. I have more to offer now, have a gift to give others.

—you gave Nina a gift, even if she can't see it yet—

I leave behind the need to gather qualifications, evidence that I know. Now I know. It's enough to be.

Rosemary:

I call the picture Metamorphosis.

A green line of ups and downs. At the beginning I was the one who didn't put my symbol on the group space—I wasn't ready. I was different at the beginning—and at the end! Sticking to my 'no'. Then, here, was a difficult patch. I needed to sit still, let things go on around me before I could get up.

Here, I'm sliding down, when Geraldine left. A shock.

Here I worried: will I do the portfolio?—all that work.

The last two weeks, the lowest slump; the heavy burden of giving Nina a 'no'. And then I come up—and I'm flying! Through the dark—up, to fly! The only way forward.

Heather:

This hut is about my roots in South Africa. I had to work on that before I could move on. Then I moved up and I got bigger. Here I'm blossoming. A wonderful spiritual blossoming. Here's a bench—I can sit and reflect! I'm really orange—my true colour. Sometimes—here—I show pink—not true to myself.

Kim:

Here I am, meeting Liesl at the interview. And now, this bundle, I've fetched away from the course. I can hold my head up high. Be in tattered shorts and barefoot—it doesn't matter.

Liesl has an image of a fan. She folds one out of pale green paper. She holds it at the base. Allowing others to unfold. As she holds it, it turns up at the edges, becomes a shell.
The feminine principle.
The womb container.
Enacting the process—says it all!

I ask for

Feedback on the course content and structure
Kim would like more time for supervision—doesn't know what she'd relinquish for it.
Support groups could be suggested. (But weren't. The 4-6 group made such provision).
Rosemary has drawn a symbolic gift for everyone.
Heather gives everyone a wooden bead—each different, part of a chain.

Exercise 31—Angel Cards
Liesl puts down angel cards—face down.
(Angel cards—from Findhorn: a pack of small cards, each with a different human quality. These can be used in a variety of ways—for individuals and groups, to meditate, intuit, focus.)
The angel card may be the quality needed to solve a problem; to make a decision, to know the way forward.
Each student picks the one she feels drawn to.

Rosemary: Forgiveness.
She forgives herself for having been so hard on herself in the past.
Heather: Honesty.
She is honest—aims to declare her spirituality more openly, honestly.
Dawn: Gratitude.
She can see the good things in her life now—and is grateful.
Kim: Spontaneity.

From being in her head, critical, to trusting herself to be spontaneous, creative, in the moment.

Marianne: Surrender.

To surrender the black cloud of self doubt, to surrender herself to what is. To be.

Wendy: Communication.

More able to be level, congruent, in her inter-personal transactions.

Liesl: Freedom

The course is about allowing others their freedom. And her freedom of a summer holiday ahead.

Time to celebrate—with wine, and food, to bring our time together to a close. A comprehensive year, ending on a well-earned high—whilst acknowledging the ups and downs of the journey and the sadness of the ending.

Dawn adds:

'These sessions have helped to bring to the surface many things that I have to work on. Negative thought patterns such as:

"If I worked harder I could make things better."

"You are good at helping out others, but no-one is going to help you."

"Even if you ask, no-one will listen," etc. etc.

All the things that say to me "don't take risks, it won't be worth it." This course has been a journey down a street named 'Risk' for me. I have learned to express my true feelings and deal with the consequences of doing so. I have learned to use criticism constructively. I have learned to listen to my needs and ask for what I want, as well as say no to what I don't want. Most important of all, I have learnt to tell the difference.

The group sessions and reading haven't done all this exclusively of course, and the process is by no means over, but they have acted as an important catalyst in my personal development. I have learned to take risks again and feel good enough about myself that the outcome hardly matters. The gain is always in the doing. I am beginning to find my way again and have hopefully developed some skills and techniques which will enable me to be as effective a catalyst for my clients. In the words of Carl Rogers, I can truly say that I have experienced 'a quiet revolution'. Thank you all.'

Marianne adds:

'I must admit to a certain amount of scepticism in the early days. "Are people making things up?" "laying it on thick"—Sometimes nothing relevant appears. The King's New Suit of Clothes.

Being in an all women-group is a new experience for me. I think it enabled me to relax and be more open, nice not to have that dominant factor. It has felt like a safe place. 'A student' was a dominant factor: it was a relief when she left but I had regrets too, more confrontation could have been good for me!

I have often felt churned up, ill at ease after sessions. Bringing up things I didn't particularly want to address at this moment in time.

Sometimes I've felt I haven't given it my all but I think I did what I was able to at this time. It will be good to have Wednesday afternoons back again, more time, one less commitment.

I have gained more than I realise. How to be more assertive. New tools for working with. What being client-centred *really* is about.'

Comments

This session, of all, was the hardest to report: the facts are there, yes, but how to convey the mood, the feelings of trust, closeness, caring, sense of achievement in the year gone by, the feelings of sadness and loss that this group will not meet again.

In offering these courses where trust and intimacy do develop, and with it so much learning and awareness, the cost for me, as tutor, is the sense of loss with each ending. Overall, a price worth paying.

I know the ending of the course is not the end; some students will join the association, some do the post-certificate year, some will take the work, the learning elsewhere. Great. *And* I mustn't rescue myself, acknowledge that *this* group has come to an end, allow myself to grieve its loss; a group of women with whom I shared much love, pain, joy and moments of magic. I am enriched through knowing them.

Each year I gain much learning for myself, fuelling my enthusiasm and commitment as I continue with my work.

'When the best leader's work is done, the people say: we did it ourselves.'

Lao Tzu

Application

Any last meeting of any group.

Course Comment

On recording the year, I realise that much has—inevitably—been left out—what we said and did and felt. And yet, overall, I believe the three terms have demonstrated in a very real way much of the effectiveness of the person-centred approach, of image-making, and of bringing the person-centred approach to art—thus: person-centred art therapy. The scope is wide, be it educational, therapeutic—groups, ones—in short, wherever persons need to develop. That which the students learned, was self-discovered. Now they can adapt and implement their learning in other settings.

I suspect that reading about the student's self-discovered learning, though once-removed from the experience, might have more impact than the reading of a more academic tome, justifying, I trust, the format of this book.

Now, in turn, the reader might reinforce, adapt and apply relevantly the insights gained.

> 'I watch you watching, I see you seeing, and through this second sight, as it were, I give these essential things a new clarity and freshness.'
>
> Four wise men—Tournier

> 'What we call the beginning is often the end and to make an end is to make a beginning. The end is what we start from.'
>
> T.S. Eliot—Little Gidding

APPENDIX I

One year on.
Students were invited to comment:
(1) What, since leaving the course, they might be doing differently at work as a result of the course.
(2) And how they might have changed as a person as a result of the course.

Here are their responses:

From Heather:

(1) We all have a few experiences in life that move us forward—this course has been one of them for me. It was the tool I needed at the right time.

At an *Adolescent Mental Health and Family Therapy Unit* I find there are three areas that I now approach differently.

Firstly in the mornings in the classroom I work from first negotiating a contract with each pupil on admission, as to what *they* wish to achieve and we work together on how to achieve this. We frequently revise and update this as change occurs. (If they wish to 'do nothing', well we look and discuss this—'nothing' never lasts!)

Secondly I use P.C. art therapy in a weekly group and also individually with the young people and may even use it spontaneously if someone is stuck and receptive to that way of working.

Thirdly the course has affected my inter-relationship with the multi-disciplinary staff team. I try to be person-centred and find this has clarified many issues for me as to what my role is as teacher and art therapy facilitator in the unit. Sometimes it has oiled wheels, sometimes others have found me uncomfortable to live with.

(2) I feel more confident, I feel as if I have an approach that suits me and from which I can move. The art therapy itself has satisfied something creative in me, stimulated the 'explorer' and that is often a joyful experience. I have and am refining my awareness of others and myself which constantly opens fascinating insights—I listen and observe with greater interest. I feel I have a greater understanding of myself and am more tolerant and kinder to myself.

I am becoming the tool which I struggled to acquire—it does need constant sharpening!

From Jo:
I left the group because of pressure of work and family traumas. Even so, I was able to integrate my learning from the course into *my work as a photo therapist and artist.* It was particularly useful as part of my initial coming to terms with being diagnosed as having Lymphatic Leukaemia, where I was able to visualise my feelings and explore them as part of my self healing process.
love, Jo
Sadly, Jo died in June 1992.
I am indebted to David, Jo's husband, for making available to me her pictures.

From Kim:
(1) I began using person-centred art therapy *in a school with two groups of nine and ten year olds.* All the children were chosen because their teachers were concerned about lack of concentration, withdrawal, social difficulties, family difficulties or disruption in the classroom. I emphasised repeatedly that I did *not* modify behaviour, but enabled the children to express and get in touch with feelings in a safe place through using the person-centred approach of empathising, accepting and being congruent.

I discovered how valuable was the *process* of creating and how the children used the materials to act out experiences and emotions. I saw how rich was their symbolic world and how creatively they used it to heal themselves. I learnt, more than anything, that they *knew* what they needed most and how to get it from me if only I made myself totally available in a non-directive way.

Since then I have moved on to another school where I spent a year working with nine, five, six and seven year olds on a weekly basis mainly in small groups but with some individual sessions. As well as paints, pencils, etc., I provided sand, water, clay, puppets, building materials, a wendy house and dressing-up clothes. Also as part of my development process I had fortnightly supervision sessions with an experienced p.c. art therapist. Again it was the children who have been my greatest teachers. If I made an inappropriate intervention they withdrew or told me I was wrong. If I spent too much time with one child they told me. It was up to me to hear it. I was less afraid to mirror what I saw was being presented. This made me focus on what I find the hardest aspect of the p.c. approach —being congruent.

Finally, I have begun to work with adults at a treatment centre for problem drinkers. Here I am in a group setting in a small room with limited resources. I realised that any planning (which initially I had tried to do) was useless therapeutically. How did I, however wise, know where the clients were before even entering the room? This realisation meant that I needed to become familiar with a wide range of activities fitting a wide range of circumstances, and offer them spontaneously. It also meant that at times I was very scared, and, having taken the risk, very pleased.

I can now note my pacing, and develop my abilities to remain congruent. This is not an easy way to work but it certainly empowers the client and encourages growth and potential.

(2) During the last session of the course I stated that had I met myself as I was the previous September I would not have recognised myself.

Now, a year later, I feel more than ever that my comment was true in that I have learnt to be clear about who I am and to be skilled at communicating my personal needs and professional aims in a positive, precise and constructive manner.

My voice, physically, has changed—I actually speak louder. I walk taller. I dress in a brighter, more confident mode.

The essence of me has not changed; I have just been enabled to trust what I feel and believe I know. I am far less afraid of taking risks—which has opened a new world of infinite possibilities.

To risk has been my greatest learning point on the course. Risking has been extremely painful as well as joyful, causing alienation as well as deepening relationships.

I am constantly consolidating the experience of the course.

From Marianne:

(1) *In my work with people with drink problems* I introduce art therapy when they are stuck, verbally going over the same ground again and again. It lifts people out of the trench and puts a new perspective on the problem.

I am soon to introduce it to a support group for friends and family of drinkers for the same reason.

I was delighted to obtain a grant from the Alcohol Education and Research Council for a research project. For this I decided to start a weekly group for men from a residential rehabilitation centre...There was enormous enjoyment in the creative process. One week, based on the request of group members, I took each person individually and looked at the work they had done...and I think they enjoyed this session the most.

(2) I have become more aware of the power I and each of us has within to influence and effect change that is desired or necessary without being controlling. Therefore I am becoming more assertive.

From Mary:
(1) Since doing the course I initiate and run person-centred art therapy groups at a *community centre for the terminally ill, for those needing respite care and for those needing rehabilitation,* with much greater confidence.

(2) The course did help me insofar as triggering me to look at my feelings particularly related to my childhood and also death. This was helped by our group process and sharing (tapping into myself) but greatly by putting images down on paper and relating the visual aspect to the internal side—the whole process of P.C.T.A. helped with this.

I feel I have grown in confidence.

From Rosemary:
(1) I have managed to obtain part-time work for every day of the week in the area of *mental handicap,* and I have also retained my voluntary job in *mental illness.*

Whenever I have had a difficulty with a client, a stuckness, a not knowing which exercise to use, or how to lead a mentally disabled client to an insight on a complex subject, I have always found it useful to revert to the basic training given on the person-centred model, i.e. stick with what the client brings, let go of the need to control. I have never known it to fail, in fact if I can be strong enough to trust, I have found that the results exceed my highest expectations. It is the hardest thing in the world to be strong enough to let go of that control, to be free of the feeling that I know better than the client what their problem is, and where they need to go. I find that I try too hard sometimes to fulfil their expectations of myself as their guide, leader or teacher. Especially in mentally handicapped people, they have learned to look to professionals for authority, to be told what to do always, and I find that often I am accepting and getting carried away with this usurped power.

I am probably less directive and controlling in both mental illness and mental handicap. More likely to provide space, time, materials and listening ears rather than set a task.

(2) I have learned to approve of and love myself, which has enabled me to share myself with my clients and to love them unconditionally. I learned to understand my own internal processes so that I recognised them when they threatened to impose on clients as interpretations. I am so much less critical and defensive since doing the course. It changed my life for the better.

From Wendy:

(1) One year on—I am still co-ordinating the *Winchester Cancer Support Group* as I was during the Course.

I have found that many of the counselling skills and dealing with group problems I experienced during the course have been a great help and I have been able to use what I learnt in our cancer group—such as getting the members to make decisions about how the group should be run. Listening skills and reflecting back have been particularly useful. In other words, using the person-centred approach where I can in the group.

Also, I go to a new Day Hospice in Basingstoke to offer person-centred art therapy. I go on a voluntary basis one morning a week. I listen and suggest they might like to have a go with crayons and paper, and see what comes up for them. Then we talk about it. One lady particularly has opened up and talked about herself and her anxieties. She says that since coming to the centre her life has changed—to be with caring people, to be listened to. I felt I could claim a part of that.

(2) During last year's course the fact that I needed more time to paint and that this was important came up many times and that the spiritual side was of great importance to me too. I am painting more...I know that when I can really let go the colour will come through that can be used as a form of healing—your course enforced my belief that I have to work on this and the freedom to do this is of vital importance.

APPENDIX II

Some past course students, too, were asked:
  (1) What they might be doing differently at work as a result of the course;
  (2) And how might they have changed as a person as a result of the course.

Their replies are grouped according to their work setting:
  (1) Education
  (2) Health
  (3) Self-help groups
  (4) Therapy/counselling
  (5) Management

---

(1) Education

Jane writes:
(1) Work setting: Islington Sixth Form Centre.

Now using P.CAT in individual work with students and it's particularly effective in helping them to express, understand and work through deep feelings, e.g. of grief or anger.

Also using P.CAT with groups of students—it is astonishingly effective. It provides an easy vehicle for expressing and sharing feelings which I know would not be possible with this age-range in a group based on talking only.

Also in my occasional work with deaf social workers, imaging through P.CAT provides evidence we can share which transcends the restrictions of communicating through interpreters only.

(2) P.CAT has enabled me to identify blocks to getting in touch with my intuition. Recently it has provided a sudden breakthrough to my creative self and to my latent ability of second sight.

Kairen writes:
(1) I feel that I am responding and interacting with others (teachers, pupils, parents and other professionals) much more openly and much more 'straight-forwardly'. I find it easier to

communicate exactly what I feel I have to say and less need to 'couch' things in jargon. I am working with pupils with emotional and behaviour difficulties. I often have to deal with a lot of 'side-issues'—since the course I have been able to see and...act much more clearly, positively and directly.

(2) I am more aware of my own 'emotional baggage', the stuff I project onto others—this is making me more objective and also more able to feel what really matters at the time rather than feeling and acting on left-over stuff from other times and situations. I feel much more satisfied by all areas of my life—even those with difficulties because I can see them for what they are, maybe grow through them. I feel much more positively and generously to others because I am being this way to myself. I am realising that although so many of my needs went unrecognised, unacknowledged in my past I actually don't have to work on that base any more and I now have the power (well—I always had it but I can see that now) to go towards meeting my needs and then the needs of others if I choose.

Lindsay writes:
Impact on my work now
I feel especially lucky, since leaving the course I have had the opportunity as tutor on a counselling course to use art work in experiental groups. This has been tremendous. The response from other women is very reassuring. The women appear to find imaging a safe and interesting way of beginning to get back in contact with hopes and fears about themselves and their lives. For many, art work has had the effect of freeing them, to look at their own needs for—(perhaps the first time)—a long time. I think that some of the women have wanted to take the experience further and have attended some of your day courses! (which they have enjoyed).

Margaret writes:
(1) During the course, I ran several PCAT workshops for teachers as part of a Counselling Skills course offered by a colleague. I realised then how much I enjoyed working with groups of adults; each time I was surprised anew by the wealth of insights and the willingness to share what happened.

At present I am running a series of six workshops for teachers from primary, secondary, and special schools. There are eight people in the group, seven women and one man, and they are all feeling really stressed. The comment most frequently made is, 'How wonderful to have something which is just for me!'

I am also offering, as part of a wider scheme to offer support to school staffs, 'one-off' workshops to teachers in their own schools.

I use the skills acquired on the course to enrich my work with emotionally and behaviourally disturbed children. As many of the children do not have the vocabulary to express feelings, PCAT provides them, and me, with a glimpse into what may be going on for them.

(2) Attending one-day workshops, before I started the training course, enabled me to explore my feelings about my changing role with regard to my parents; imaging helped me to come to terms with their increasing age and frailty, and to identify my own needs. During the training course and in the post-certificate year which followed, I was enabled, in a very supportive setting, to face the many losses of the past few years, to express my anger and sadness and to realise some of my anxieties and fears.

Since the course I have continued to grieve but in a healthier way. I am aware not only of my feelings but of those of others and this has enriched my relationships with those around me. I am MUCH better at looking after myself!

Sally writes:
(1) I was counselling children using a variety of techniques such as Rogerian, Gestalt and T.A. I now use the art as a fundamental part of the counselling. I find it works very well with children—particularly those who aren't very verbal or who aren't in touch with their feelings. I work as a teacher and part time counsellor in a school for disabled pupils.

(2) I found the experience of P.C.A.T. very rich and exciting. I felt that issues were revealed to me through the art which wouldn't necessarily have come to the surface through just talking (because I have more control over this process). It also made me aware of the healing capacity of our own images and metaphors.

Veronica writes:
(1) Work setting (A): Individual Teaching Service

> Pupils, in general, have emotional/psychological problems; have difficulty in expressing themselves especially in writing etc. Are loathe to express themselves because they feel they lack the necessary writing skills; do not want to appear as failures—therefore they withdraw from the risk of trying...

Since participating in the course and working with such pupils, I have found that offering individuals an 'Art Therapy' exercise has opened a door to them by offering an alternative for self expression in a free and unthreatening manner and has led to self confidence in their self expression, through drawing and relating. I now use various exercises as acceptable means of communication for individual pupils, introducing the offer as 'another' way of putting what they feel down without the 'bother of thinking about words, spellings etc.'

I also now offer the possibility of illustrating their written work (often stunted) by the addition of an exercise. This develops into an enjoyable and more full participation of a sharing—and tangible 'evidence' of success becomes available to the pupil.

Work setting (B): Small Parish Group/children receiving Religious instruction

I now relate to such a group in quite a different way. During the first session I introduce the exercise of drawing an image of how they feel in this new place, group etc, hoping to give the opportunity of each getting in touch with themselves—not, as previously, giving and extracting 'knowledge'.

Also, in introducing for e.g. the theme of 'Reconciliation' I would now invite them to draw an image of

(a) when someone said 'sorry' to them,

(b) when they said 'sorry' to someone,

and they would share how they felt.

I have found this approach refreshing both from the point of view of my own approach to this work and to their participation and inter-relation. I feel the group gets at a different level.

(2) I have changed very much in 'awareness', e.g. I am very much more aware of the occasions when I draw back and refrain from making assumptions/judgements about persons, situations etc.

I am much more 'person-conscious' and have learnt to respect the freedom of 'the other' more.

I tend to negotiate much more and I hope to be consulted, too.

The value of the IMAGE plays a great part in my life, e.g. I can ask myself—'what image floats up for me in this particular situation'...and reflect on it.

More accepting about the reality about what life offers and being able to respond in ways such as 'rituals'. I used to be rather cynical about this! My trust and openness have grown.

---

(2) Health

Anna writes:

(1) I now have, I feel, an invaluable tool in approaching the emotional/psychological problems of many of the children I assess. My work setting is the Child Development Centre, Charing Cross Hospital, London W6. I see children who are in mainstream schools who are referred for perceptual/motor problems which often it transpires, have emotional overlay or longstanding related problems. I have also been enabled to work with troubled parents whose difficulties are compounding those of their children. I am immensely grateful for the skills gained on the course and now wonder how I managed without them, and some of my most satisfying times this year have come from using this approach.

(2) The course brought into focus many issues it has been useful to explore further. Whenever I have the opportunity to work with images for myself I feel illuminated by the process. I feel more in touch with the power of non verbal expression and the directness of this way of working. It's knowing now something from the inside in addition to acknowledging it intellectually as a potent process.

George writes:

(1) Work setting: College of Nursing & Mid-wifery.
    Position: Senior Educational Manager (Mental health Nursing)
    Within the college I am now teaching the basic principles of P.C. art therapy to psychiatric/mental health student nurses,

qualified paediatric nurses (RSCN), student general nurses (RGN) and also to volunteer counsellors outside of my work situation. I am constantly talking to and encouraging my colleagues to work in a more person-centred way.

(2) I'm sure I function much more spontaneously and intuitively inside and outside of work. My wife says I'm more aware of her/others. I feel I'm more self-aware and a 'fuller' person.

Janet writes:

(1) (Adults with cerebral palsy). Whilst working in a residential centre I gave clients more time and did not feel tempted to jump in and get things done at my speed.

At work now (Day Centre for adults with mental health problems) I am able to listen better and enable people to help themselves by not advising, but by allowing them time to see for themselves.

(2) My husband tells me I listen more, he is able to say things more he wouldn't have before and that my temper has improved! I do try to allow people to take the lead more within the family and try to let my young children express themselves more freely, creatively and emotionally. I feel more confident now in some situations.

I am more self aware.

Linda writes:

(1) Adult education art teaching in mainstream provision and as an agency working within other organisations: Greenwich District Hospital (geriatric and stroke patients), Age Concern (elderly mentally frail) and Greenwich 'MIND' Centre.

In these different settings according to the needs of the respective groups I'm aware of using the person-centre approach to counsel elderly students and stroke patients where art therapy has also been useful, by helping to develop a more independent approach towards students own work and to incorporate person-centred art therapy skills as an occasional input as part of an on-going art workshop for people with mental health problems who also want to develop and practice their technical skills in drawing and painting.

(2) I've gained insight into a way of tapping into my own feelings and suppressed or forgotten memories of events that had not been resolved. This has allowed me to alter my perception of those events and has allowed me to accept them. I listen more carefully to my children and let them know that I've heard them and express my feelings honestly to them.

Megan writes:

(1) I work in a Day Centre for the Elderly as an O/T Technician. As a result of the Course I run a Therapeutic Art Group using the skills learnt. In this setting I am able to encourage patients to work through areas of psychological discomfort. These may include bereavement reactions and/or issues pertaining to loss of independence, poor self esteem, accepting and coping with changed circumstances, etc.

(2) Since attending the Course, I have discovered I need to understand myself before I can begin to understand others. It has enabled me to mature in this area. It has also helped me to build on improving my confidence, which for me was a weak area.

Merle writes:

(1) Volunteer Visitor for a Hospice Homecare Service for five years.

The major difference was learning to LISTEN—to myself, patients and their carers and the professional team at Hospice. Contrary to previous behaviour (when I appeared to accept unfair blame easily) listening clearly, reflecting back and, particularly, learning to be responsible for myself while not shouldering others' problems, seems to have confused my superiors.

As a result of the exercises for my portfolio (armed with further P.C. Art Therapy) I may pursue a new direction facilitating fellow artists in working through longstanding 'blocks'.

Coping with a group situation is easier than before.

(2) Personal work during the course enabled me to clear out a large amount of unsolved 'dross', leaving me with more inner confidence, calmer, able to deal more in perspective with difficult situations. I 'rescue' less—have more personal space as a result.

Sally writes:
(1) As a result of the learning gained from the course I now use art in my work not only for relaxation and fun but am able to facilitate the psychiatric patients I work with to understand what their worries may mean for them in a caring and person-centred way.

(2) I have become more accepting both of myself and others, am a better listener and have more courage to be honest with myself and other people.

Sue writes:
(1) I work as a Clinical Specialist Nurse in a community setting. Since completing the course I have used the PCAT skills with the children I come in contact with. Either children with life threatening illness or children who have been or will become bereaved. Colleagues now used me as a resource to them.
   I have also been involved in growth groups for staff.

(2) I have become far more accepting of myself and my abilities.
   I take risks more easily.
   I trust others to take risks too; I'm very rarely a rescuer or a blamer now.
   I take responsibility for myself and feel good about it.

---

(3) Self-help groups

Annette writes:
(1) I have a stronger belief and commitment to student centred learning and the value of the process!

(2) As a person I feel I know myself much better through my participation in the course. It classified issues. I can more clearly see the work I have to do. It having deepened my knowledge of myself gives me confidence in the process and its potential for others and myself. Changing is hard.
   The reading list which I munched on throughout the course intensified and confirmed my experience. The course for me was very important and helped my *change*.

Hilary writes:

(1) Having *met* more of myself through the course, I am able to *offer* more of myself. To work in a person-centred manner is something to believe in and aim for.

I'm certainly more able to be real, and so I hope and believe am more trustworthy in my interactions.

(2) My inner and outer worlds have drawn closer together through my valuing of the symbolic. I feel fuller in a brighter, clearer, deeper, darker and more mysterious landscape. Also happier! (for having tested out through imaging, more of myself. I might not have dared elsewhere/other ways.)

---

(4) Therapy/counselling

Angie writes:

(1) Using the client-centred approach better because I am now more familiar and fully appreciate it.

As well as offering counselling, now using art therapy as an extra 'tool' within the sessions.

(Worksetting—working with families in voluntary sector. Referred families from Soc. Services).

(2) Through the experiential learning, although at times painful, I embarked on a journey of self and discovered the real me. I'll continue on this voyage until the end of time. The journey of life. On my voyage I threw away my rubber ring in order to swim and have quit rescuing!

Brenda writes:

(1) I'm working in Day Centre for the elderly and as trainer and counsellor in Bereavement Counselling. The main change in the way I work is in being constantly aware of the person-centred model of counselling and finding it more and more the best way to move people forward. It is the first time in my years of counselling training that I feel I now have a model. The overall two years has given me a confidence in believing that any non-verbal tool—art, clay, collage, postcards etc, can become a vehicle for aiding change and that art is particularly effective—as long as the client can overcome resistance!

(2) I have gained confidence both through learning a new skill and because of various insights gained during our exercises. I have a more realistic understanding of my own needs and limits and value myself more.

Ginnie writes:

(1) At the Family Welfare Association, where I am a counsellor, I now use visualisation techniques and art exercises when appropriate, and work with more awareness of the person centred approach.

(2) The processes of the course have enabled me to be more conscious of my own feelings and therefore to feel more integrated. As so often seems to be the case, I was on the course, at a time when it was a most valuable thing for me to be doing.

June writes:

(1) Work setting: Co-ordination of Jewish Bereavement Counselling Service.

Plan and run group supervision sessions. Bereavement Counsellor.

I allow the counsellors and clients to be more person-centred. Very aware of taking power away when using interpretation. I now try to give power back to counsellors and clients as much as possible. Have used art therapy in counselling and in group supervision. I am aware of the power of imaging and have used technique in counselling.

Am very aware of example set by Liesl when running groups. Boundaries decided upon by the group were strictly adhered to and I am using this in my group sessions.

(2) Use of images allowed me to share my feelings immediately in the group. As a result I feel more confident in groups and am more able to state my needs. Through Liesl's example I saw how I had to take responsibility for myself and not to blame others for my own inadequacies. The P.C. approach made me feel 'very safe' and I felt my words were important. No-one judged or interpreted what I was saying. I was accepted for what I was and this gave me a great deal of confidence.

Laura writes:

(1) My approach to my clients and their feelings has changed: I listen more and now can hear them. I feel more confident in my ability.
Using imagery brings the feelings forward, is direct.

(2) Effected my outlook and perception of myself in the world in general, and gave me more confidence in myself and in my abilities.

Lily writes:

(1) I have been using imaging and art therapy in my counselling skills training groups, with individual clients, with families during therapy, and with couples in marital difficulties.

(2) Become more person-centred in my work and in my private life. More aware of self and of others' feelings. Course highlighted and illuminated and also confirmed beliefs and ideas I had held previously.

Mary writes:

(1) With my clients, incorporating art therapy more by using 'spot imaging' and then drawing the image. Also understanding the content of drawings more and allowing clients to speak for themselves.

(2) I think I've become more congruent, understand the difficulties caused by interpretation and have become more creative generally.

Maxine writes:

(1) Private work setting/group facilitator at University:
Encouraging use of non-verbal communication through the use of art and then looking at what has been produced in a person-centred way. Emphasis is much more on what the person tells me—not to interpret—that's probably the biggest difference.
I try to see if I can use visualisation and art with individuals and groups whenever the opportunity arises, and if it doesn't—I try to create opportunity for it!

(2) I've got in touch with my creative side—and I enjoy taking my experience from your course to others. I'm a lot more confident with 'ART' and its powerful, liberating experience.

Sibylle writes: (from Zurich)
(1) Here, as promised, a small summary of my work:
   I've finished my training with Liesl in summer 86, moving back home to Switzerland soon afterwards. Since then I've opened up my own practice for person-centred-art therapy, also counselling and developing teams in helping professions. The non-direktiv and non-interpretiv approche and skills applied in this spezial arttherapy have turned out to be very successful indeed.

   In the meantime I've also become a trainer at the statecollege for socialwork with children and youngsters from damaged or broken families. Here too I use the skills learnt at Liesl's to develop the students selfawarness, creativity and selfesteem and to grow empathy, congurence and acceptance towards others. We do a lot of co-counselling with paintings and drawings which is ever so important working with children.

   The troublesome business of having to mark the students work I solved with introducing selfassessment and assessment of each other on a regular basis. After the first scary moments the students felt that all trainers should use this method of assessment and organised a big meeting including the principal of the college. The collegeboard is now seriously deskussing this matter!

   As a boardmember of the swiss-association for counsellors and as co-editor of their professional-bulletin I've taken the chance to introduce the approach and skills of person-centred art therapy to my colleagues, suggesting how they could use it in their counselling-setting. I've received a lot of positive feedback for these artikles.

   Looking into the future I've started to think about the possibility of giving courses myself for the professionals in the counselling field of Zurich.

(2) What ever happens I will always remain deeply grateful to Liesl and her person-centred-arttherapy, which opend the dor and heart not just to my inner self but to all of menkind—I've become a scolar of life itself!

Personal experiences of the course
It was important for me to just try to be more creative with my own life experience. Imaging brought back memories and gave me the possibility of doing something in a different way. I found it exciting and frightening because it put me so quickly in touch with sadness. Often things became more part of my awareness after the session—feelings once I had left seemed more powerful though I didn't always know what these were about. I spent a lot of time crying. This was helpful—since I am aware of lots of sadness in me. I gained in confidence from the course—feedback from other members was an important aspect of this. In particular I felt more able to take in and be helped by positive feedback—I guess I felt relieved; it may be that this is truly at the heart of the person-centred approach—and that this came through to me on the course. The course held me at a time when I was feeling particularly vulnerable—imaging made it safe for me to acknowledge what was happening—and to share what I wanted. It felt challenging and safe.

---

(5) Management
Wendy writes:

(1) *Commercial working environment—mainly managers*
Doing differently—person centred approach—holding off a bit more with me, the expert.
trusting in them finding their way.
taking on more one-to-one counselling.

(2) *Personal*: In many ways—things still help—coming up and falling into place—leaving me feeling more relaxed.
—increasingly aware of the darker side—I know there are more things to be worked on—but I don't yet know when this time will come—but I feel more courage to be able to cope with them.

APPENDIX III

Some work settings of some past students
Acute psychiatry
Adult education—one to one counselling
Adults with learning difficulties
Alcohol counselling
Art therapist
Assertiveness trainer
Astrological counsellor
Bereavement counselling
Cancer support
Careers guidance
Centre for the deaf
Child development centre
Child protection
Child psychiatry
Church counselling
Colour therapist
Community mental health centre
Counselling
Dance therapy
Drug dependency unit
Drug prevention
Education
Educational and mental health
Elderly with mental health problems
Family centre
Head teacher—special school
HIV—worker
Hospice worker
Hypnotherapy
Individual teaching service
Information technology teacher
Lecturer—psychology
Management consultant
Mental health—counselling
Mental health day hospital
MIND counsellor
Minister of religion
Nursery teacher
Nursing
Occupational therapy

Parents group
Pastoral head
Personnel management
Peripatetic teacher
Physically handicapped
Primary school
Psychiatric staff nurse
Psychotherapist
Rape crisis counsellor
Refugee worker
Relate counsellor
Remedial teacher
Residential unit—adolescents
School for physically disabled pupils
Social services—counselling
Speech & dyslexia therapy clinic
Student counselling
Teacher—autistic children
Teacher—emotionally disturbed children
Teaching adults in prison
Tutor, F.E.
V.S.O. trainer
Welfare officer
Women's centre
Women's refuge
Young persons unit
Youth club
Youth worker

BIBLIOGRAPHY

Adamson, Edward. *Art as Healing*. Coventure Ltd.

Axline, Virginia. *Dibs in Search of Self*. Pelican Books.

Bettelheim, Bruno. *The Use of Enchantment*. Peregrine Books.

Edwards, Betty. *Drawing on the Right Side of the Brain*. Fontana Books.

Kramer, Edith. *Art as Therapy with Children*. Feder.

Liebmann, Marian. *Art Therapy for Groups*. Routledge.

Mearns and Thorne. *Person-Centred Counselling in Action*. Sage.

Miller, Alice. *The Drama of being a Child*. Virago.

Milner, Marion. *On not being able to Paint*. Heinemann.

Oaklander, Violet. *Windows on our Children*. Real People Press.

Rogers, Carl. *Client-Centred Therapy*. Constable.

Rogers, Carl. *On Personal Power: Inner Strength and its Revolutionary Impact*. Constable.

Rogers, Carl. *A Way of being*. Houghton Mifflin Company.

Rhyne, Janie. *The Gestalt Art Experience*. Brooks/Cole.

Satir, Virginia. *Making Contact*. Celestial Arts.

Stephens, John. *Awareness*. Real People Press.